Common Skin

Thomas F. Poyı

MB, BS, MRCP, MRCGP, DRC

General Practitioner
Queens Park Medical Centre
Stockton-on-Tees, UK

**Blackwell
Science**

© 2000 by
Blackwell Science Ltd
Editorial Offices:
Osney Mead, Oxford OX2 0EL
25 John Street, London WC1N 2BL
23 Ainslie Place, Edinburgh EH3 6AJ
350 Main Street, Malden
  MA 02148-5018, USA
54 University Street, Carlton
  Victoria 3053, Australia
10, rue Casimir Delavigne
  75006 Paris, France

Other Editorial Offices:
Blackwell Wissenschafts-Verlag GmbH
Kurfürstendamm 57
10707 Berlin, Germany

Blackwell Science KK
MG Kodenmacho Building
7–10 Kodenmacho Nihombashi
Chuo-ku, Tokyo 104, Japan

The right of the Author to be
identified as the Author of this Work
has been asserted in accordance
with the Copyright, Designs and
Patents Act 1988.

First published 2000

Set by Excel Typesetters Co., Hong Kong
Printed and bound in Spain by Hostench sa,
Barcelona

The Blackwell Science logo is a
trade mark of Blackwell Science Ltd,
registered at the United Kingdom
Trade Marks Registry

DISTRIBUTORS
Marston Book Services Ltd
PO Box 269
Abingdon, Oxon OX14 4YN
(Orders: Tel: 01235 465500
         Fax: 01235 465555)

USA
Blackwell Science, Inc.
Commerce Place
350 Main Street
Malden, MA 02148-5018
(Orders: Tel: 800 759 6102
         781 388 8250
         Fax: 781 388 8255)

Canada
Login Brothers Book Company
324 Saulteaux Crescent
Winnipeg, Manitoba R3J 3T2
(Orders: Tel: 204 837 2987)

Austrialia
Blackwell Science Pty Ltd
54 University Street
Carlton, Victoria 3053
(Orders: Tel: 3 9347 0300
         Fax: 3 9347 5001)

A catalogue record for this title
is available from the British Library and
the Library of Congress

ISBN 0-632-05134-5

For further information on
Blackwell Science, visit our website:
www.blackwell-science.com

Contents

Preface, vii

1 The spectrum of disease, 1

2 How to get the diagnosis right, 14

3 Rashes on the face, 22

4 Scalp problems, 34

5 Generalized rashes, 37

6 Flexural rashes, 68

7 Hands and feet, 76

8 Abnormal nails, 84

9 Lumps and bumps, 87

10 Investigations, measurements and referrals, 99

11 Managing common skin diseases, 108

12 Management of acne and other facial rashes, 109

13 Management of eczema, 117

14 Management of psoriasis, 125

15 Management of flexural, hair and nail problems, 130

16 Urticaria and rashes without surface scale, 133

17 Management of skin infections, 135

18 Management of leg ulcers, 143

19 Formulations, 145

20 Specific therapies in detail, 150

21 The team approach, 162

22 Self-help, 165

References, 167

Index, 171

Preface

This book is designed to help all those who deal with the common dermatological problems in their daily practice. Skin disease has a major impact on people's lives. Despite 15% of consultations in general practice being for diseases of the skin, the average GP receives little or no dermatological teaching [1]. The primary healthcare team should be able to cope with the long-term management of most patients with chronic skin problems.

This book aims to be a user-friendly guide to common dermatological problems. It is intended to present dermatology as a practical subject. Chapters 1–2 set the scene on what is likely, what to ask and where to look for clues, Chapters 3–8 are designed to aid the diagnosis of rashes at different sites. While common diseases are dealt with in detail, rarer conditions are also mentioned; the reader may then refer to more comprehensive literature.

Chapters 12–22 guide one through the implementation of appropriate therapy. The treatment of common conditions is covered first, then individual therapies. By the end of the book you are nearly an expert! No attempt is made to cover minor surgery; there are already some excellent small books in existence by finer wielders of the scalpel than I [2,3].

Thomas Poyner

The spectrum of disease

Although there are a vast number of dermatological conditions, a small number lead to the majority of inappropriate referrals [4]. The common conditions one comes across in primary care are:
- acne
- atopic eczema
- contact dermatitis and other forms of eczema
- psoriasis
- viral warts and other skin infections
- benign and malignant skin tumours
- leg ulceration.

These common diseases should form the basis of any core curriculum of either undergraduate or postgraduate education for those involved in primary care. Brief notes on these and other common skin problems are given in this chapter.

Common skin conditions

Acne
- a disease of the pilosebaceous glands
- patients have seborrhoea
- vast majority of teenagers affected, with 15% having clinically significant disease
- can affect other age groups, e.g. 7% of those aged 28–40
- caused by abnormal response to physiological levels of androgens
- rash consists of blackheads, whiteheads, papules, pustules and nodules
- rash—face and trunk
- can produce irreversible scarring
- differential diagnoses—rosacea, perioral dermatitis and seborrhoeic eczema

> **Rosacea**
> - common in middle age
> - cause unknown, may be result of solar damage or a vascular problem
> - *Helicobacter* and the *Demodex* mite have been implicated
> - rash—papules, pustules on erythematous background
> - affects cruciate distribution of the face
> - flushing—worse with spices and alcohol
> - rash does not have blackheads and whiteheads

Eczema

> **Eczema**
> - the most common reason for a scaly rash
> - terms eczema and dermatitis are synonymous
> - term eczema is derived from the Greek 'to boil over'
> - eczema can present in different ways depending on its stage and type
> - stages—can be acute or chronic
> - types—atopic, seborrhoeic, discoid and contact

Different types of eczema		
Exogenous	Endogenous	Unclassified
Irritant contact	Atopic	Asteatotic
Allergic contact	Seborrhoeic	Lichen simplex
Photodermatitis	Discoid	Juvenile plantar dermatosis

Adapted with permission from *Exploring Eczema: a Distance Learning Package* (1995). Haymarket Publishing Services, London.

Atopic eczema
- affects up to 15% of children and 10% of adults
- accounts for 30% of dermatological consultations in primary care
- one of the atopic conditions—asthma, eczema and hay fever
- combination of genetic and environmental factors
- house dust mite is a common allergen and soap an irritant
- infection is a common reason for exacerbations
- initial presentation is as non-specific eruption with facial involvement
- localizes to the flexures at elbows and knees
- patients have a facial pallor
- rash is itchy and a child can be fretful
- associated with dry skin
- in adults the rash can be similar to children, or present just as a hand dermatitis
- common differential diagnoses—seborrhoeic eczema and psoriasis

Contact dermatitis

There are two types of contact dermatitis, contact irritant and contact allergic dermatitis. The hands are a common site of contact dermatitis.

Contact irritant eczema
- some patients are more susceptible, e.g. those with atopic conditions or dry skin
- common sites are hands and nappy area
- one has to consider the strength of the irritant and the frequency of exposure
- there are weak and strong irritants, soap is an example of a weak irritant
- differential diagnoses—other eczemas and psoriasis

CHAPTER 1

Contact allergic eczema
- contact allergic eczema occurs at the point of contact with the allergen (Fig. 1)
- can get a rash at other more distant sites
- nickel in jewellery is most common, affecting approximately 10% of females
- can be caused by topical medication, e.g. neomycin
- one must have a high index of suspicion
- do not forget hobbies and occupations
- patch testing needed to confirm diagnosis
- differential diagnoses—other eczemas, fungal infections and psoriasis

Common causes of contact allergic dermatitis	
Allergen	Found in
Nickel	Jewellery
Lanolin	Creams
Colophony	Sticking plasters

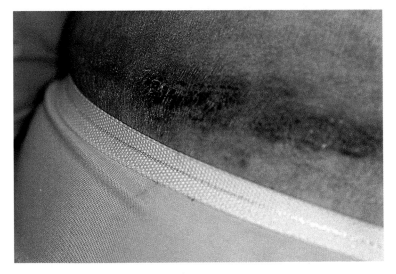

Fig. 1 Allergic contact dermatitis—elastic.

Other eczemas

Infantile seborrhoeic eczema
- cases usually present before 12 weeks of age
- happy baby with nappy rash and scaly scalp
- does resolve but some go on to develop atopic eczema

Adult seborrhoeic eczema
- occurs at sites where sebaceous glands are plentiful
- sebum excretion is normal
- *Pityrosporum* yeast plays some part and may be the cause
- patients have a greasy scaly scalp
- mildest form is dandruff
- widespread disease can be associated with AIDS
- can involve eyebrows, ears and nasolabial folds
- may involve the presternal area and flexures
- differential diagnoses include atopic eczema, psoriasis and Darier's disease

Discoid eczema
- often develops in middle age
- rash is very itchy
- presents as discrete coin-shaped patches on the trunk and limbs
- surface covered in a crust or scale
- secondary bacterial infection is common
- differential diagnoses include psoriasis and tinea corporis

Pompholyx
- can be associated with increased sweating
- occasionally associated with nickel hypersensitivity
- more common in summer months
- presents as a symmetrical erythematous rash with vesicles
- vesicles can coalesce to form bullae
- occurs on the palms, sides of the digits and soles
- secondary infection is common
- patients get recurrent attacks
- differential diagnoses—contact allergic dermatitis and localized pustular psoriasis

Lichen simplex
- very itchy plaque
- scaly surface with accentuated skin markings
- found on neck or lower legs
- can become pigmented
- differential diagnoses—Bowen's disease, psoriasis and tinea

Asteatotic eczema
- a form of irritant dermatitis
- affects the elderly in the winter
- presents as a dry skin with crazy paving appearance
- common site—lower legs
- differential diagnoses—other eczemas

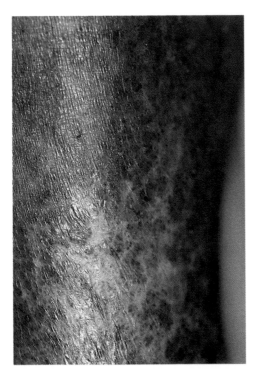

Fig. 2 Venous eczema.

Venous eczema (also called stasis eczema and varicose eczema) (Fig. 2)
- associated with venous disease
- only occurs on lower legs
- oedema and pigmentation may be present
- beware of contact allergic dermatitis to medications
- differential diagnoses—other eczemas

Darier's disease (Fig. 3)
- autosomal dominant
- rash—pinkish brown papules with greasy scale
- distribution—rather seborrhoeic pattern: face, behind the ears and chest
- palms and soles—pits/punctate keratoses
- nails—longitudinal ridges

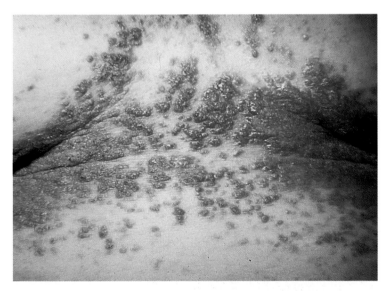

Fig. 3 Darier's disease.

Psoriasis and common differential diagnoses

Psoriasis
- common chronic inflammatory skin disorder affecting 2% of population
- genetic susceptibility and often a family history
- environmental factors include streptococcal infections, trauma and stress
- tobacco, alcohol and stress may be detrimental
- presents as red well-defined plaques with silvery scale
- usual sites are scalp, elbows, knees and lower back
- guttate psoriasis presents as 'rain drop like' small scaly papules
- most cases improve with sunlight but a few deteriorate
- nails—onycholysis, pitting and salmon patches
- differential diagnoses—seborrhoeic eczema, discoid eczema, lichen planus, pityriasis rosea, pityriasis rubra pilaris, urticaria and drug rashes

---

Lichen planus
- can be idiopathic or caused by drugs
- very itchy rash on limbs and genitalia
- red/violaceous flat-topped papules
- scaly surface with white streaks—Wickham's striae
- produces lace-like pattern in mouth
- leaves pigmentation as it clears
- nails—grooves, pitting and nail loss
- can cause scarring alopecia

Pityriasis rosea
- cause unknown, possibly viral
- usually a young person
- initial large scaly patch—herald patch
- pink scaly oval patches
- fir tree distribution of rash following lines of ribs
- lasts approximately 6 weeks

Pityriasis rubra pilaris
- aetiology unknown
- rash—extensive red scaly patches with follicular plugging
- feature—islands of 'normal' skin
- palms and soles—thickened smooth and yellow

Urticaria
- can be acute or chronic
- rash consists of weals
- individual lesions are transient, lasting less than 24 h
- weals are raised itchy lesions caused by dermal oedema
- acute is caused by foods, e.g. shellfish and strawberries, or drugs, e.g. penicillin
- chronic is of at least 3 months' duration and is usually idiopathic
- salicylates can both cause and exacerbate urticaria
- urticaria can be associated with angioedema
- angioedema—acute swelling of the lips and eyelids

Drug eruptions
- drug reactions can produce any type of rash
- urticaria—penicillin, NSAIDs and captopril
- maculopapular—penicillin and phenothiazines
- pigmentation—oral contraceptives, dapsone and gold
- photosensitivity—tetracyclines, thiazides and sulphonamides
- fixed drug eruptions—laxatives

Viral warts and other skin infections

Viral warts (Fig. 4)
- caused by the human papilloma virus
- different subtypes associated with different clinical presentations
- clinical presentations include common, plane, plantar and genital warts
- warts spontaneously resolve
- differential diagnoses—molluscum contagiosum and malignant lesion

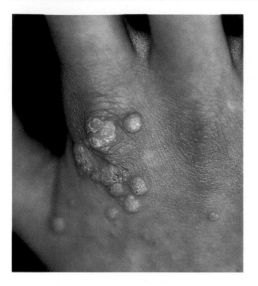

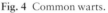

Fig. 4 Common warts.

Molluscum contagiosum
- caused by a pox virus
- common in children and teenagers, especially atopics
- presents as dome-shaped papules
- usually multiple grouped lesions
- lesions have a punctum and contain cheesy material
- eczema may surround the lesions

Impetigo
- caused by *Staphylococcus aureus* or *Streptococcus pyogenes*
- frequently on the face of children
- yellow crust and sometimes blisters
- rapidly spreads and is contagious

Tinea pedis
- caused by infection with dermatophyte fungi
- produces erythema and scale
- itchy rash on feet, especially between toes
- can infect the toe nails—thickened, deformed and onycholysis
- differential diagnoses—juvenile plantar dermatosis and pitted keratolysis

Scabies
- severe nocturnal itch
- affects family members
- scaly papular rash on trunk and limbs
- burrows found on the sides/between fingers
- burrows are linear tracts
- papules on the male penis
- differential diagnoses—eczemas and lichen planus

Benign and malignant skin tumours

Seborrhoeic warts are common and patients are often relieved to be informed that they are benign. Common malignant skin tumours are basal and squamous cell carcinomas, and these tend to be associated with prolonged sun exposure. Melanoma tends to affect a younger age group and be associated with acute episodes of sunburn.

Seborrhoeic warts
- common benign tumour
- numbers increase with age and sun exposure
- are uniform in shape and colour
- have a 'stuck on' appearance
- have a greasy feel
- have a cribriform scaly surface

Dermatofibromas
- benign small pigmented tumour
- do not increase in size over time
- uniform shape and firm feel
- usual site—lower limbs
- dimple on squeezing

Banal naevi
- are uniform in shape and colour
- do not change rapidly in size
- have a regular edge
- are symmetrical
- differential diagnoses—seborrhoeic warts and melanoma

Angiomas
- caused by benign overgrowth of blood vessels
- smooth dome-shaped red lesions
- sharp margin between lesion and normal skin
- differential diagnosis—melanoma

Basal cell carcinomas
- common on face or back of elderly patients
- usually nodular or cystic
- slowly increasing in size
- raised rolled edge, often easier to see on stretching the lesion
- pearly with telangiectasia
- can be pigmented
- differential diagnoses—sebaceous gland hyperplasia, cellular naevi and keloids

Actinic keratoses
- caused by chronic solar damage
- found on the bald heads and backs of hands of elderly patients
- red scaly rough areas
- most either static or resolve, a few progress to squamous cell carcinoma
- if any substance to lesion one needs to exclude squamous cell carcinoma

Squamous cell carcinomas
- occurs on sun-exposed sites
- presents as a papule or nodule
- can ulcerate and have a crust over lesion
- can develop from an actinic keratosis
- differential diagnoses—actinic keratosis, viral wart, keloid and keratoacanthoma

Melanomas
- associated with sunburn in childhood
- risk factors—fair skin, red hair, blue eyes and burn easily
- often superficial spreading or nodular lesions
- some develop from benign naevi, especially atypical and large congenital naevi
- rapid change in size and shape
- irregular colour
- irregular edge
- differential diagnoses—banal naevi, seborrhoeic warts

Leg ulceration

Leg ulcers are a cause of both morbidity to the patient and expense to health services. Many leg ulcers could be better managed and healed in primary care.

Leg ulceration
- approximately 2% of a practice population has leg ulceration at some time
- 80% are venous in origin
- need to treat with compression bandaging after excluding arterial disease
- other aetiologies include arterial, diabetic or mixed pathology

How to get the diagnosis right

In one study only 47% of referrals contained the correct diagnosis, one should therefore ask what we can do to improve this [5]? Dermatology is very much a visual subject and most, if not all, of the clues to the correct diagnosis are before us. It does no harm to have a quick glance at the rash, as the diagnosis may be obvious, and some rashes are 'once seen, never forgotten'. However, if not, one needs to do some detective work and proceed to take a history.

History

Simple history for a skin disease
- where did the rash start?
- where has it spread to?
- what was its appearance and has this changed?
- does it itch or weep?
- how does it bother you?
- have you or your family ever had this rash before?
- what are your occupation and hobbies?
- what medication are you taking?
- what treatments have you used?
- what seems to make the rash better or worse?

Where and when did the rash start and where has it spread to? Has its character changed? What treatment if any has been used? This is important, as treatment can modify the clinical picture of many rashes. If a fungal rash is misdiagnosed and then inappropriately treated with a topical steroid, the inflammation is reduced and the picture becomes atypical; this is known as tinea incognito. If a rash is asymmetrical unilateral erythematous and scaly, or has a raised edge, consider the possibility of a fungal aetiology.

Itch

Do inquire about itch; if all the family members have developed severe nocturnal itch, scabies is highly likely. A localized itchy patch on the lower leg or back of the neck is likely to be lichen simplex. Multiple very itchy scaly lesions suggests lichen planus. The presence of excoriations (scratch marks) suggests an itchy skin. Children with atopic eczema often exhibit them.

Family history

Family history is often helpful, and something on which the GP can be an expert! Frequently there is a family history of either psoriasis or the atopic conditions, such as eczema, asthma and hay fever.

'It's me job doctor!'

One next needs to determine the patient's occupation, e.g. hairdressers are renowned for having hand dermatitis. Patients with atopic eczema should have, but frequently have not had, advice regarding avoiding occupations which involve frequent skin irritation. There is evidence that people with acne find it harder to find employment [6]. Patients with acne have difficulty entering the armed forces as working in a hot climate is detrimental. Travel and living abroad can predispose to skin cancer, e.g. living or working in Australia or the Gulf. No history is complete without inquiring about pastimes and hobbies, e.g. gardeners can develop a whole host of rashes from plants.

'It's me nerves doctor!'

Many patients still associate skin disease as being caused by anxiety. While this is not true many skin conditions, such as psoriasis and seborrhoeic dermatitis, can deteriorate at times of stress. One should always inquire about a patient's psychological well-being; some patients can tolerate skin problems better than others. Many patients receive help and support from their families and friends, while others experience rejection. Patients with problems such as acne can pose a real suicide risk.

Those vices

Increased alcohol consumption is associated with a flare of plaque psoriasis, while smoking is incriminated in localized pustular psoriasis. The skin manifestations of other vices are occasionally encountered. The author remembers seeing a case of secondary syphilis in a chap who had been to Holland and visited more than the bulb fields over a weekend!

The notes and computer screen

It is worth looking in the notes or 'at the screen' (with new VDU technology) for a previous entry which might give a clue to the correct diagnosis. A record of a prescription for penicillin may give the diagnosis for a morbilliform rash. Previous entries regarding sneezing and wheezing point to a diagnosis of atopic eczema. An old maxim is that for an unexplained exanthem in a child a viral aetiology is likely, while for the elderly either a drug reaction or malignancy should be high on the list of possibilities.

Examination

The rash

We need to examine the lesion or rash. This should be done in a good light, preferably daylight. A simple hand lens enables the surface of lesions to be inspected, and adds a certain level of style to the consultation! The number of lesions is helpful; a localized scaly patch could possibly be ringworm or Bowen's disease while a more generalized scaly rash would suggest psoriasis or eczema. The site of the rash can be a big clue; acne occurs on the face and back, while pompholyx occurs on the hands and feet. One needs to decide what lesions are present in the rash and whether they are discrete or coalesce.

Stand back and look at the sites and distribution

Next it is worth standing back and looking at a rash; one can get too close initially to see the wood for the trees. The sites involved are a great help to diagnosis, e.g. atopic eczema involves the flexures, while psoriasis is seen on elbows and knees. It is worth observing to see if the rash spares certain areas, e.g. photosensitive rashes spare under the chin and behind the ears. Sometimes it's worth viewing a rash from a different angle; suddenly one recognizes the clinical picture. If all else fails ask the patient what they think it is!

Is it symmetrical?

It is worth observing if the rash is symmetrical; if it is this suggests that it is probably endogenous, e.g. psoriasis. If a rash is asymmetrical or unilateral then external causation should be considered, e.g. tinea, or a contact allergic dermatitis.

Bet on the favourite

Do think 'what is the most likely diagnosis'. Common things are common, and the atypical presentation of a common disease is more likely than some extremely rare condition. It is worth having a mental picture of what a typical patient with each common dermatosis looks like.

Use the examination room occasionally!

Do look at sites other than those the patient has mentioned. Using the examination room reduces the time lost waiting for the patient to undress, and gives one the chance to glance at this book for guidance.

If you think the rash on the elbows could be psoriasis then look at the scalp and nails for evidence of this disease. If you suspect lichen planus, look for the fine white lace-like pattern in the mouth. The arrangement of lesions is helpful. A rash may be linear, e.g. herpes zoster, or clustered on the lower leg, e.g. insect bites, or can occur at sites of trauma and scars; this is Koebner's phenomenon (Fig. 5).

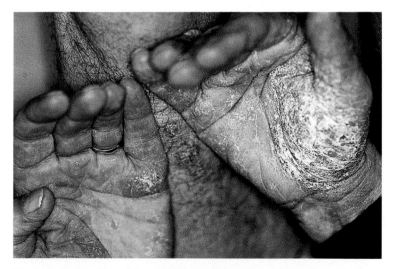

Fig. 5 Koebner's phenomenon—psoriasis after a burn on the hands.

Koebner's phenomenon is associated with:
- psoriasis
- lichen planus
- seborrhoeic eczema
- plane warts.

Getting to know the language

One needs to decide what lesions are present in a rash. Looking at the skin's surface, redness is termed *erythema*. There may be *exudate*, e.g. acute eczema, and that exudate which accumulates and dries forms *crusts*, e.g. impetigo. Surface *scale* may be present, e.g. psoriasis, or there may be *fissures*, e.g. contact irritant hand eczema. The skin may be thickened (*lichenification*) along with *excoriations* from scratching.

Sign	Description
Erythema	Redness of the skin
Crust	Accumulated dry exudate
Lichenification	Area of thickened skin
Excoriation	Scratched skin

A partial break in the skin is an *erosion* which can occur with rupture of a blister. A complete break is an *ulcer*, e.g. varicose ulcer.

Sign	Description
Fissure	Crack in the skin
Erosion	Partial break in the epidermis
Ulcer	Complete break in the epidermis

A small flat area of altered colour is a *macule* while a larger area is a *patch*, e.g. a patch of eczema, and a large elevated area is a *plaque*, e.g. a plaque of psoriasis. An area of dermal oedema is known as a *weal*, e.g. urticaria.

Sign	Description
Macule	Small area of altered skin < 1 cm
Patch	Larger circumscribed area of skin >1 cm
Plaque	Large raised area >2 cm
Weal	Transient elevated area

A small raised spot is a *papule* and a larger area is a *nodule*, e.g. acne. A small blister is a *vesicle*, e.g. herpes simplex, and a larger one is a *bulla*, e.g. pemphigoid.

Sign	Description
Papule	Small raised area <1cm
Nodule	Larger raised area >1cm
Vesicle	Small fluid-filled lesion <1cm
Bulla	Fluid-filled lesion >1cm

A small lesion containing pus is a *pustule*, e.g. rosacea. A *furuncle* is localized bacterial infection of a hair follicle, and if a group coalesce then a *carbuncle* is formed. A localized collection of pus in a cavity is an *abscess* and an infection of the nail fold is a *paronychia*.

Sign	Description
Pustule	Small pus-containing lesion <1 cm
Abscess	Pus-containing lesion >1 cm
Furuncle	Infection of a hair follicle
Carbuncle	A collection of furuncles

Play dermatological aerobics, pick, scratch, squeeze and stretch

One can scratch a rash to see if it is scaly, suggesting epidermal change. Dermatologists are great scratchers! Psoriasis has large silvery scales with a well-defined edge while ringworm has fine scale and a raised border. Pityriasis versicolor is scaly but vitiligo is not. Picking or removing the crust from a lesion makes the diagnosis easier, e.g. basal cell carcinoma. Rashes, such as urticaria and granuloma annulare, have no surface change.

A seborrhoeic wart has an uneven surface. When the skin is stretched a basal cell carcinoma becomes more obvious. A dermatofibroma feels firm and the skin dimples when it is squeezed. Only by palpating acne can one discover the extent of deep nodules. Palpation enables one to feel for atrophy associated with certain conditions. One should test the temperature of the skin using the back of the hand. A cellulitic leg feels much warmer than the healthy limb.

The colour—dermatological rainbows

Erythema is caused by vasodilatation; this blanches on pressure. Purpura is different in that there is extravasation of blood so it does not blanch on pressure. Melanin produces brown pigmentation. Some rashes are associated with specific colours (well, at least in other textbooks if not in real life); these colours include:

- violaceous with lichen planus
- heliotrope discoloration with dermatomyositis.

Sign	Description
Erythema	Redness of the skin
Purpura	Blood outside vessels
Telangiectasia	Dilated small blood vessels

Diascopy can easily be performed using a glass slide pressed on the skin. It causes blanching of vascular lesions enabling one to see the original colour.

The border, or over the edge!

The edge of the rash often aids diagnosis. Psoriasis has a well-defined edge, such that one could almost trace it, while eczema has a much more ill-defined edge. Tinea has a raised edge with central clearing. The edge of granuloma annulare is similarly raised, but there is no surface change. Circumscribed means there is a distinct edge between the rash and normal tissues.

The shape of the lesion—Picasso at work!

The lesions of discoid eczema are coin shaped, and those of tinea corporis can form a ring. Burrows are synonymous with scabies. Any unusual shape would raise the possibility of a rash being artefactual or a contact allergic dermatitis. Some tumours are pedunculated.

Arrangement of lesions

Lesions may remain discrete with normal skin between them. They may be grouped in one area or they may be unilateral. The discrete lesions may be disseminated all over the body or they may become confluent to form a generalized rash.

Vive la différence

General practice differs from hospital consultancy; one can easily bring the patient back and have another look. The rash might just be evolving; a solitary scaly patch may herald the arrival of the classical rash of pityriasis rosea 3 days later. One can always photograph a mole which appears benign if one still has a lingering doubt at the first consultation and arrange a review.

How to look professional

A magnifying glass can be useful, especially when viewing possible skin malignancy. A bonus is to press the glass against a purpuric lesion to demonstrate that it does not blanch. For the experts there is a dermatoscope!

Well, it all helps

Now at least one can describe the rash and, if nothing else, the referral letters have gone from economy to club class!

3 Rashes on the face

When trying to make a diagnosis, knowing the age of the patient is a good starting point. This is usually not too difficult to guess, but if all else fails one can look at the notes. A two year old with a facial and flexural rash probably has atopic eczema, while a 15 year old with pimples on the face and back most likely has acne.

Children

If a baby has a scaly scalp and nappy rash, he or she has infantile seborrhoeic eczema (Fig. 6) unless proved otherwise. This rash can also involve the trunk and flexures. Atopic eczema, by comparison, starts with a scaly erythematous rash on the face and a rather nondescript rash on the trunk. It then goes on to localize in the cubital and popliteal fossae. Atopic eczema spares the napkin area as the increased moisture is beneficial. Infantile seborrhoeic eczema presents around 2 months of age, which is slightly earlier than atopic eczema.

The infant with eczema		
	Atopic eczema	Infantile seborrhoeic ezcema
Onset	After 3 months	Often before 3 months
Duration	Continues	Resolves
General state	Often fretful	Happy
Site	Face initially	Face, scalp and nappy area

Adapted with permission from *Exploring Eczema: a Distance Learning Package* (1995). Haymarket Publishing Services, London.

Children frequently present with hypopigmented slightly scaly patches on their cheeks. This is pityriasis alba and is associated with atopic eczema.

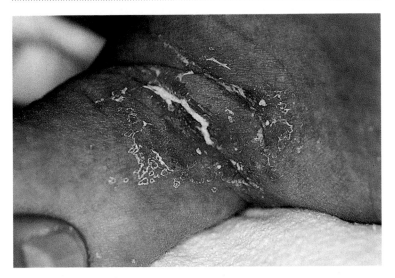

Fig. 6 Infantile seborrhoeic eczemas.

Localized lesions
Yellow crusted lesions on the face suggest the diagnosis of impetigo (Fig. 7). There are both bullous and non-bullous forms. Herpes simplex presents as painful vesicles.

Rashes involving the ears
Atopic eczema causes fissures on the ears, while seborrhoeic eczema causes erythema and scaling around the ears. Pruritic papules and vesicles develop on the ears of young boys with the solar-induced condition of juvenile spring eruption.

Adults with red faces

One needs to look at the type of rash and its distribution (Fig. 8). One should not forget to take a history of sun exposure and the use of cosmetics and toiletries. The predominant lesion and presence or absence of surface change are important.

The swollen red face
Angioedema presents as swelling of the lips and eyelids. It can be

23

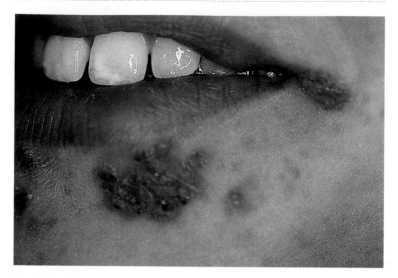

Fig. 7 Impetigo.

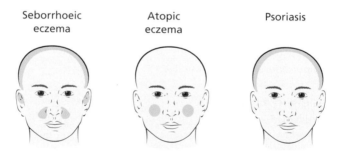

Fig. 8 Diagnosing facial rashes: commonly affected areas.

associated with most forms of urticaria. If there is any problem with respiration caused by obstruction then urgent hospital referral is indicated. Acute contact allergic dermatitis can present as a swollen red face. Airborne allergens, such as cement powder, cause a widespread symmetrical rash while topical allergens, such as a cream, only produce a rash at the site of contact.

The hot red face
Erysipelas presents as a well-demarcated asymmetrical facial ery-

thema. Looking at the patient from a tangent sometimes aids the diagnosis. There is oedema of the tissues but no surface change. The tissues are hot and tender to touch and the patient is often pyrexial and toxic. This is an infection which is situated in the dermis and is caused by *Streptococcus pyogenes*.

The red face with spots

With acne and rosacea there are papules and pustules but no scaling. Acne commonly affects the face, chest and back (Fig. 9). In acne there are also open comedones (whiteheads) and closed comedones (blackheads) (Fig. 10). Stretching the skin can make comedones more obvious. Acne can also cause nodules and scarring, with palpation often aiding their diagnosis. The patient with rosacea has papules and pustules on an erythematous background (Fig. 11). Inappropriate use of topical steroids can produce a similar result.

Front

Back

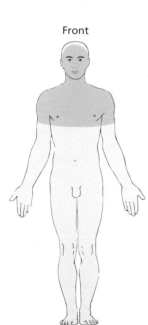
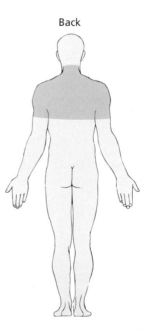

Fig. 9 Acne: commonly affected areas.

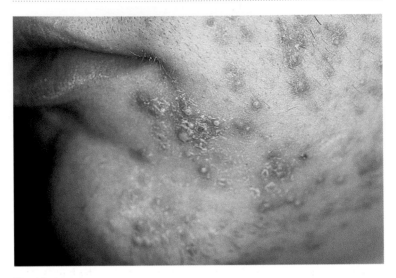

Fig. 10 Acne.

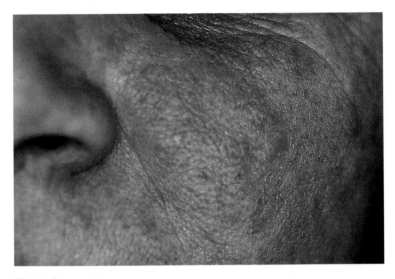

Fig. 11 Rosacea.

How to differentiate between acne and rosacea		
Feature	Acne	Rosacea
Comedones	Present	Absent
Erythema	Variable	Present
Flushing	Absent	Present
Onset	Second or third decade	Later
Papules and pustules	Present	Present

The rash of perioral dermatitis (Fig. 12) is similar to that of rosacea in containing both papules and pustules. However, their distributions are different:

• rosacea has a cruciate facial distribution; and
• perioral dermatitis involves the perioral area.

One should be suspicious of polymorphic light eruption if a rash develops on light-exposed areas in a young female. The hands, face and neck may be affected with itchy papules and vesicles. The rash may, or may not be eczematous in nature.

The nosy patient		
Disease	Presentation	Appearance
Rosacea	Rhinophyma (Fig. 13)	Enlarged with hyperplasia of sebaceous gland
Sarcoid	Lupus pernio	Deep purple plaques

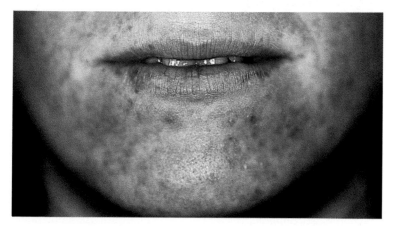

Fig. 12 Perioral dermatitis.

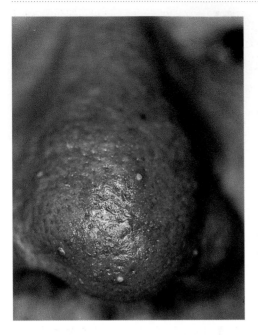

Fig. 13 Rhinophyma.

The red face with vesicles

The usual cause is a herpes simplex type 1 infection. Repeated attacks of cold sores are common, often occurring on the same site, such as the lip or face, and presenting as painful vesicles (Fig. 14). Respiratory infections and ultraviolet light can act as triggers. It is worth advising sufferers about using a high-factor lip protection. Herpetic lesions can crop up at various sites and if there is any doubt it is advisable to take a viral swab.

Septic lesions in the beard area

A folliculitis is an infection of the opening of hair follicles. The usual site is the male beard area, although thighs and buttocks can also be involved. Sycosis is a subacute infection of the whole hair follicle (Fig. 15). On the male beard area papules and pustules form which can coalesce.

The red scaly face

The two most common causes of a scaly facial rash are seborrhoeic eczema and psoriasis. The family history often helps discriminate

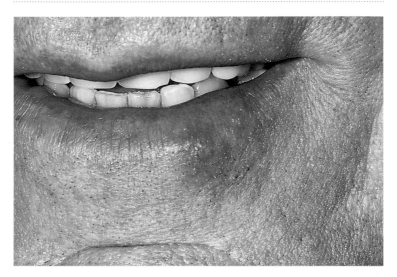

Fig. 14 Herpes simplex.

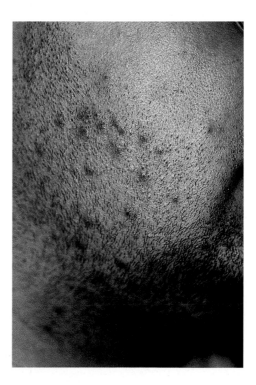

Fig. 15 Sycosis barbae.

between the two. The presence of scaly red plaques on the elbows and knees makes the diagnosis of psoriasis.

Differences between adult seborrhoeic eczema and psoriasis		
Feature	Seborrhoeic eczema	Psoriasis
Scalp	Greasy scale	Silvery scale
Trunk and limbs	Scaly petaloid rash on sternum	Plaques on trunk and limbs
Flexures	Erythema	Well-defined erythema
Nails	Normal	Deformed

   Seborrhoeic eczema presents as a greasy scaly scalp with a scaly red rash in the nasolabial folds, on the eyebrows and behind the ears (Fig. 16). Otitis externa can be caused by seborrhoeic dermatitis or a contact allergic dermatitis to a topical antibiotic, e.g. neomycin. In contrast, photodermatoses spare behind the ears and under the chin, as these areas are shaded from sunlight. Any rash which involves the face, hands and neck raises the possibility of a photodermatitis or a photo-aggravated rash.

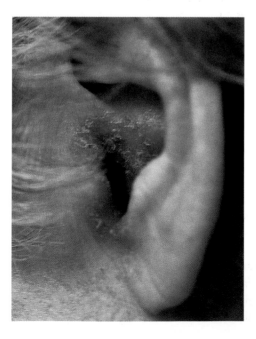

Fig. 16 Seborrhoeic eczema—ear.

The ears	
Disease	Findings
Atopic eczema	Fissures
Seborrhoeic eczema	Otitis externa
Contact allergic dermatitis to ear drops	Eczematous rash on external ear
Contact allergic dermatitis to jewellery	Eczema on lobes
Chondrodermatitis helicis nodularis	Tender skin-coloured papules
Solar keratoses	Red scaly lesions, no induration
Sarcoid	Deep purplish red colour
Juvenile spring eruption	Papules and erythema on ears

Every medical student learns about, but few see, the butterfly rash on the face associated with the joint pains and arthralgia of systemic lupus erythematosus; however, one is far more likely to come across discoid lupus erythematosus. When one sees localized red slightly scaly patches with follicular plugging one should think of discoid lupus erythematosus. Scarring can also be a feature and the rash is aggravated by sunshine. Rarely, tinea can infect the face and when it infects the neck it produces a very angry asymmetrical pustular type of rash. In this situation one should enquire about contact with animals.

Allergic contact dermatitis of the face
Rashes on the eyelids raise the suspicion of contact allergic dermatitis. Contact allergic dermatitis can occur from cosmetics, nail varnish and perfumes. Cosmetics and perfumes produce a rash at the site of contact. Nail varnish can cause a rash on the face, especially the eyelids, because the nails are brushed across these sites. Hair dye can also cause contact allergic dermatitis on the face and scalp. Plants can produce a dermatitis caused by airborne particles. An airborne allergy does not spare behind the ears or under the chin as a photosensitivity allergy does.

Rashes on sun-exposed sites
Those with red hair and fair skin are very susceptible to sunburn, e.g. Barbara (my wife!). If a patient suddenly starts becoming very sensitive to solar radiation then one should consider the possibility of a

drug-induced or -aggravated reaction: possibilities include tetracyclines, sulphonamides and thiazides. Although most patients with psoriasis improve with sunlight a few get worse. Symptoms of patients with lupus erythematosus and Darier's disease are aggravated by sunlight. It is said that UVB burns and UVA ages the skin. Some reactions are mainly caused by UVB while others are caused by UVA, which can penetrate through glass.

If a young boy presents with papules on the ears during the spring then one should suspect juvenile spring eruption, while a young female with papules, vesicles and erythema on exposed sites would be likely to have polymorphic light eruption. Elderly men can present with a very active eczematous rash on a light exposed surface—chronic actinic dermatitis.

Problems with facial pigmentation and hair

Abnormal facial pigmentation

Melasma, which is caused by increased melanin, presents as lightly pigmented symmetrical patches on the face; in females this is known as chloasma. Some cases are associated with oral contraceptives and pregnancy. Many inflammatory dermatoses can produce post-inflammatory pigmentation which resolves with time. Lentigines are areas of uniform increase in pigmentation on sun-exposed sites. Afro-Caribbean patients can develop multiple dark papules on their faces—dermatosis papulosa nigra.

The mature face

Prolonged solar exposure takes its toll on the skin, producing solar damage as well as intrinsic ageing. The skin develops a waxy appearance with wrinkles. Next time a mature outdoor worker is in your surgery look at the difference between the skin on exposed and non-exposed sites. There are uniform pigmented macules known as lentigenes (liver spots). Basal cell papillomas occur which present as uniform symmetrical scaly lesions with a rather stuck-on appearance. Senile comedones develop which are similar but larger than those of acne. Actinic keratoses present as red rough areas which are often easier to feel rather than see; the bald male's scalp is a common site.

Hirsutism

When considering if female facial hair is excessive one must consider the patient in the context of her family and racial characteristics. One does not need to investigate unless the problem is severe, of sudden onset, periods are irregular or signs of virilization are present, e.g. deepening of the voice.

Scalp problems

The scaly scalp

The common causes of a scaly scalp are seborrhoeic eczema and psoriasis (Fig. 17). Seborrhoeic dermatitis produces greasy scale whereas
that of psoriasis is silvery. With scalp psoriasis one might also find
scaly plaques on the elbows, knees and a nail deformity with pits and
onycholysis (Fig. 18). The patient with seborrhoeic dermatitis com-
plains of itchy scalp. The mildest form of seborrhoeic dermatitis is
dandruff.

The scaly scalp

Disease	Scale	Alopecia	Scarring
Seborrhoeic dermatitis	Greasy	Unusual	Absent
Psoriasis	Silvery	Unusual	Absent
Tinea	Present	Usual	Possible

Headlice

Headlice are an increasing problem, diagnosis is rarely difficult, and
perhaps this is one situation where one does not want to get too
close. The eggs are usually visible on the hairs and one can search for
live lice if one is motivated. Headlice can result in itch, impetigo and
enlarged cervical glands.

Hair loss

Patients are often anxious about any hair loss. One needs to decide if
the problem is:
• increased shedding of hair or diffuse hair loss
• localized hair loss with or without scarring.

Diffuse hair loss

A diffuse hair loss can occur following pregnancy or ill health, this

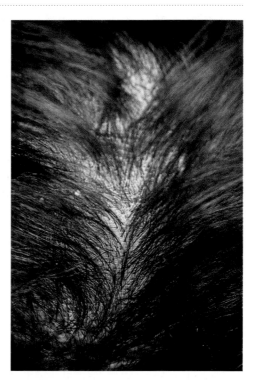

Fig. 17 Seborrhoeic
dermatitis—scalp.

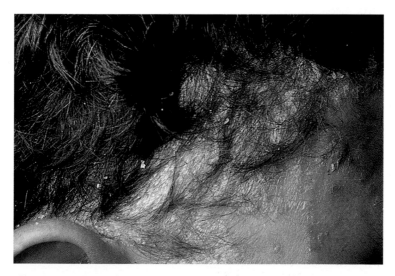

Fig. 18 Psoriasis—scalp.

being known as telogen effluvium. Other treatable causes of hair loss are iron deficiency and myxoedema. It is worth screening for these as they are treatable; many conditions are not. One should not forget that certain drugs, e.g. anticoagulants and chemotherapy can produce alopecia.

Androgenetic alopecia in males presents with frontal recession. In the female patient it is more of a diffuse loss over the vertex with preservation of the hair line. In cases of androgenetic alopecia it is always worth asking if there is a family history of this condition.

Areas of localized hair loss

Alopecia areata produces localized areas of hair loss with no surface change. It is worth asking if there is any family history of that type of problem and looking for pits on the nails. Alopecia can be associated with other autoimmune diseases, such as thyroid disease and pernicious anaemia.

Tinea capitis is usually found in children and is more common in Afro-Caribbean patients. It produces localized areas of hair loss with surface change. The clinical picture is quite variable, depending on the species of fungus, from small areas of hair loss and scale, to a very inflammatory mass known as a kerion. If alopecia is associated with scarring then one needs to exclude conditions such as:

- lichen planus
- discoid lupus erythematosus
- morphoea.

Hair loss	
Type	Features
Increased shedding	Telogen effluvium after pregnancy or ill health
Diffuse alopecia	Associated with iron deficiency and myxoedema
Androgenetic alopecia	Diffuse loss from vertex, male and female pattern
Localized loss without scarring	Alopecia areata, discrete areas, normal scalp
Localized loss with scarring	Lichen planus and discoid lupus erythematosus
Ringworm	Scaling and hair loss in children
Trichotillomania	Irregular area with residual short hairs and no scale

Generalized rashes

Dry skin

Dry skin is frequently encountered although it is probably easier to feel than see. Causes of a dry scaly skin include:

• inherited ichthyoses
• those associated with atopic eczema
• malignancy.

Dry scaly skin is common in children and is frequently associated with atopic eczema. The other common cause of dry skin is the familial ichthyoses (Fig. 19). These are a group of disorders of keratinization characterized by dryness and scaling. The most common is ichthyosis vulgaris, which is inherited as an autosomal dominant and is associated with atopic eczema [7]. The disease is mild, with dry skin and scaling but flexural sparing. There can be rough lesions which are easily felt if one rubs one's finger along the skin; these are known as keratosis pilaris. Any dryness of the skin in the elderly should raise the possibility of a malignancy, especially a lymphoma. Asteatotic eczema is another cause of dry skin, presenting on the legs of elderly patients with rather a crazy paving appearance.

Generalized itch

The cause of an itch may be obvious, such as scabies, lichen planus and urticaria. With a generalized itch without a rash one should search for signs of systemic disease and exclude:

• malignancy
• liver disease
• anaemia
• thyroid disease.

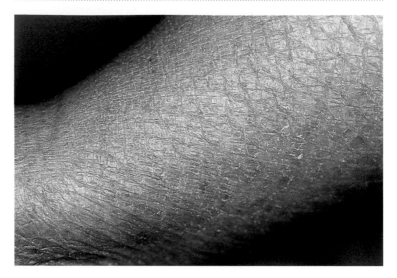

Fig. 19 A case of inherited ichthyosis.

Scaly rashes

Many rashes scale and whenever you meet a new rash your fingers should be picking away to see if it is scaly. The appearance of an eczematous rash will depend upon what stage it is in.

Eczema in different forms	
Stage	Appearance
Acute	Red with exudate, possibly with vesicles and blisters
Chronic	Dry, scaly, with lichenification and fissures

An endogenous eczema is symmetrical in nature, while the pattern of an exogenous eczema depends upon the stimulus. Examples would be the symmetrical flexural involvement of atopic eczema and the contact allergic eczema at the umbilicus from the point of contact with the nickel in a jean stud.

Trying to decide on the causation of an individual case of eczema is not always simple, as frequently it is multifactorial. An atopic indi-

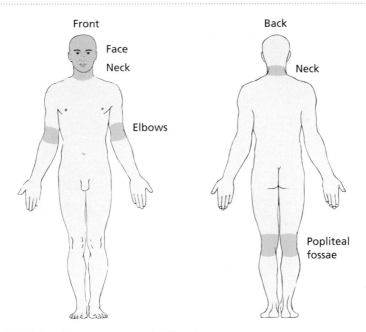

Fig. 20 Atopic eczema: commonly affected areas.

vidual is more susceptible to irritants, therefore developing an irritant eczema when others would not. Trying to unravel industrial dermatitis is a nightmare, and early referral to a dermatologist with as much information as possible is advisable.

Atopic eczema

Atopic eczema is common and is one of the atopic conditions together with asthma and hay fever. The tendency to atopic eczema is inherited, with the susceptible individual being exposed to a host of environmental triggers. Atopic eczema usually presents between the age of 3 months and 2 years. The rash starts by affecting the face, trunk and sometimes the extensor regions (Fig. 20). Eventually it involves the flexor surfaces, localizing to in front of the elbows and behind the knees (Fig. 21). There is often a very dry itchy skin.

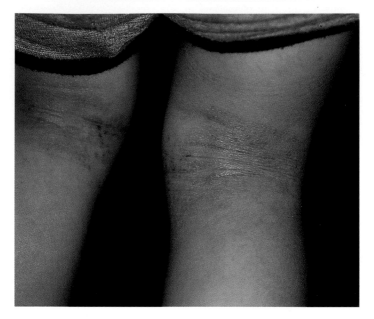

Fig. 21 Atopic eczema.

> **Diagnostic criteria for atopic eczema [8]**
> *Must have*
> • an itchy skin condition (or report of scratching or rubbing in a child)
> *Plus three or more of the following*
> • history of itchiness in the skin creases, such as folds of the elbows, behind the knees, front of the ankles or around the neck (or the cheeks in children under 4 years)
> • history of asthma or hay fever (or history of atopic disease in a first-degree relative in children under 4 years)
> • general dry skin in the past year
> • visible flexural eczema (or eczema affecting the cheeks or forehead and outer limbs in children under 4 years)
> • onset in the first two years of life (not always diagnostic in children under 4 years)

The severity of the rash fluctuates and secondary bacterial infection can easily aggravate the condition. Children with atopic eczema

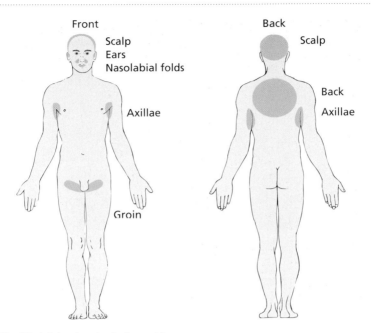

Fig. 22 Adult seborrhoeic dermatitis.

must avoid contact with people with cold sores, as herpes simplex infection produces a very severe rash known as Kaposi's varicelli-form eruption.

Adult seborrhoeic dermatitis

Seborrhoeic dermatitis presents with a scaly scalp and a rash on the face in the nasolabial folds (Fig. 22). Petalloid scaly lesions are found on the sternal area. Seborrhoeic eczema can also involve the flexures. The Pityrosporum yeast has a role in seborrhoeic dermatitis and an antifungal, such as ketoconazole, forms part of the therapy. Dandruff can be regarded as mild seborrhoeic dermatitis.

Discoid eczema

This presents as itchy coin-shaped erythematous areas covered in exudate and crust (Fig. 23). The rash is situated on the trunk and limbs, and the patient is usually middle aged. It can be difficult to dis-tinguish discoid eczema from psoriasis.

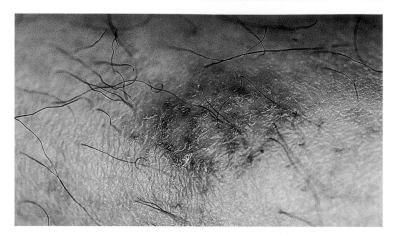

Fig. 23 Discoid eczema.

The differences between discoid eczema and psoriasis		
Feature	Psoriasis	Discoid eczema
Itch	Variable	Pronounced
Site	Elbows, knees, lumbar area	Trunk and limbs
Shape	Variable plaques	Coin-shaped
Surface	Silvery scale	Crusts, vesicles and scale
Nails	Pits and onycholysis	Normal

Psoriasis

The most common form is chronic plaque psoriasis. There are red scaly plaques on the elbows, knees and lower lumber area (Fig. 24). The plaques have a silvery scale and a well-defined edge (Fig. 25). Scaly plaques form in the scalp with hairline and ear involvement. In the flexures the rash does not have scale but presents as a red rash. The hands and feet may be scaly or covered in small reddish brown pustules. Contrary to what is often taught, psoriasis can itch. On continued scratching of the scale on a plaque it will bleed—Auspitz's sign.

Children and adolescents may develop the very small scaly lesions of guttate psoriasis (Fig. 26). This often follows a sore throat, which acts to provoke the rash in a susceptible individual. Some children go on to develop plaque psoriasis. Pityriasis rosea is a scaly eruption occurring on the trunk which sometimes causes some diagnostic difficulty. It is probably viral in aetiology.

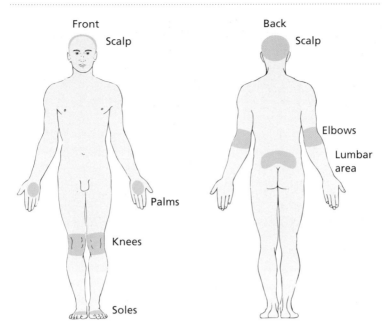

Fig. 24 Psoriasis: commonly affected areas.

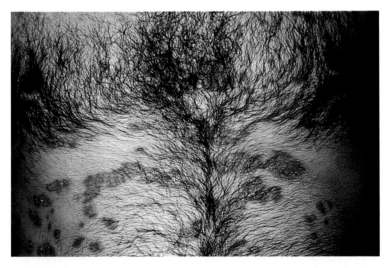

Fig. 25 Plaque psoriasis—chest.

43

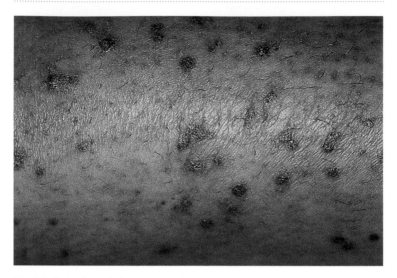

Fig. 26 Guttate psoriasis.

Scaly rashes on the trunk	
Disease	**Features**
Plaque psoriasis	Silvery scaly plaques with a well-defined edge
Guttate psoriasis	Raindrop-like scaly erythematous lesions
Lichen planus	Very itchy flat-topped violaceous papules
Pityriasis rosea	Herald patch and multiple oval pink patches
Pityriasis lichenoides	Small reddish brown scaly papules
Tinea corporis	Scaly areas with a raised edge and central clearing
Persistent superficial dermatitis	Finger-like scaly patches
Mycoses fungoides	Plaques of varying colour, atrophy and telangiectasia

Lichen planus

Lichen planus is another cause of scaly lesions on the trunk and limbs (Fig. 27). The lesions are violaceous with milky white streaks known as Wickham's striae. Patients with lichen planus report a very severe itch, while that associated with psoriasis is variable. The rash of lichen planus usually disappears within 2 years and as it resolves it leaves pigmentation.

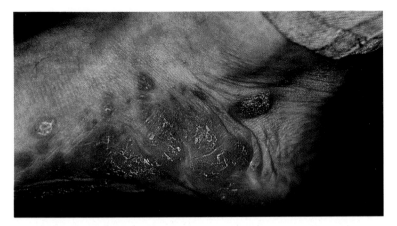

Fig. 27 Lichen planus.

Is it psoriasis or lichen planus?					
Disease	Itch	Lesions	Colour	Scale	Oral
Psoriasis	Variable	Plaques	Pink/red	Silvery	Geographical tongue
Lichen planus	Severe	Papules	Violet/red	Fine	White lace-like

Pityriasis rosea (Fig. 28)

This is probably of viral aetiology. Classically a teenager first develops the herald patch, a scaly erythematous lesion. Then, a few days later, a widespread pink scaly rash develops which follows the lines of the ribs (Fig. 29). Plaques have a collarette of scale and are in a fir tree configuration. The rash clears in approximately 6–8 weeks.

Pityriasis lichenoides

The acute form presents as red papules which go on to leave pitted scars. In the chronic form reddish-brown papules develop which become scaly and there are pigmentary changes.

Persistent superficial dermatitis

Very superficial uniform pink finger-like scaly patches develop on the trunk; only rarely is there any association with future skin malignancy.

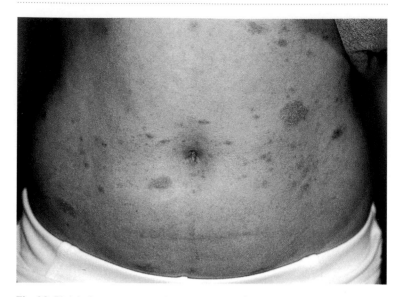

Fig. 28 Pityriasis rosea.

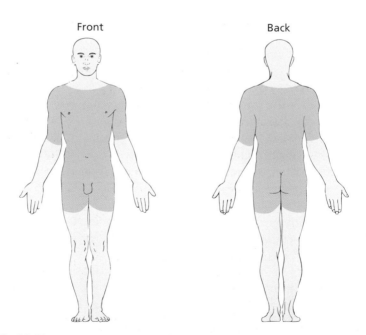

Front   Back

Fig. 29 Pityriasis rosea: commonly affected areas.

Mycosis fungoides

Mycosis fungoides is a form of lymphoma. This initially can resemble psoriasis. Well-defined patches and plaques develop which go on to display variation in size and colour. There is often atrophy, pigmentation and telangiectasia in the skin.

Causes of itchy plaques	
Cause	Appearance
Discoid eczema	Disc-shaped lesions with exudate and scale
Contact eczema	Red scaly lesion at site of contact
Lichen planus	Itchy polygonal violaceous lesions
Psoriasis	Red plaque with silvery scale and well-defined edge
Ringworm	Red annular lesions with raised edge and central clearing
Lichen simplex	Well-defined scaly plaques with increased markings

For diagnosis of scaly erythematous or symmetrical rashes the following algorithms (Figs 30 and 31) may be helpful.

Localized patches and plaques

The localized scaly plaque

The localized scaly plaque is often a cause of concern. Lichen simplex presents as a well-demarcated very itchy plaque on the lower leg or the nape of the neck. The increased skin markings aid diagnosis. The premalignant condition of Bowen's disease can simulate a localized patch of psoriasis. Tinea corporis presents as a red scaly plaque or patch with a raised border and central clearing. The rash is either circular or annular in shape. The raised border helps to distinguish this rash from psoriasis and discoid eczema.

Localized scaly plaques	
Diagnosis	Features
Lichen simplex	Well-defined thickened skin, with increased skin creases, common sites are nape of neck and lower leg
Bowen's disease	Red slightly scaly plaques often found on lower legs
Superficial BCC	Red pearly, scaly plaque with a raised edge

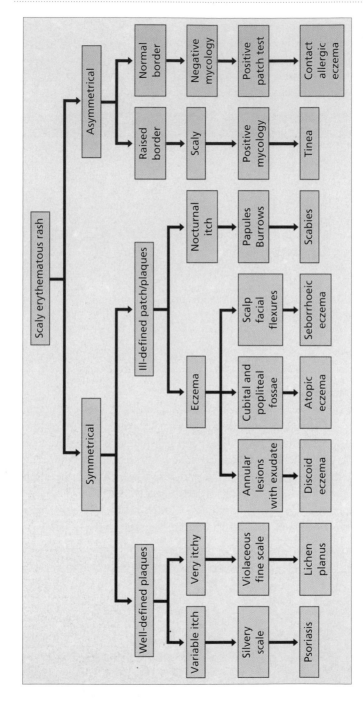

Fig. 30 The scaly erythematous rash: diagnostic algorithm.

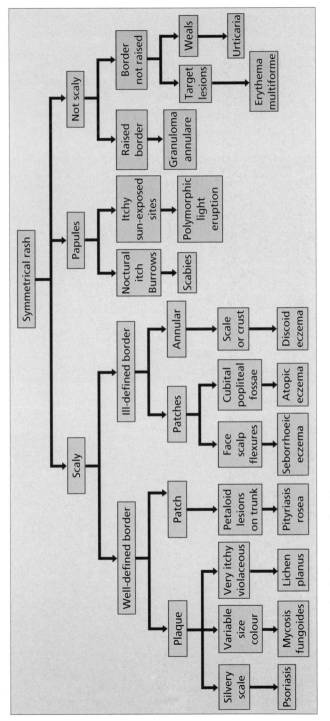

Fig. 31 The symmetrical rash: diagnostic algorithm.

49

Abnormal patches of skin

Patients are often concerned by an abnormal patch of skin. With vitiligo there is absence of pigment but no surface scale and no change in skin texture (Fig. 32). In guttate hypomelanosis there are depigmented macules on the limbs. Morphoea causes rather indurated or atrophic patches of skin with no scale (Fig. 33). The

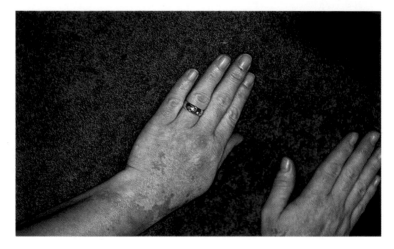

Fig. 32 Vitiligo.

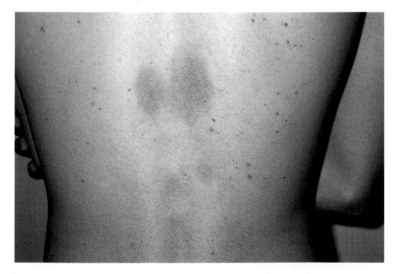

Fig. 33 Morphoea.

Pityrosporum yeast is a commensal; however, there can be an over-growth of it producing pityriasis versicolor (Fig. 34). This usually presents on the chest or back of a young adult as fawn or brown scaly patches. There is no raised border as for tinea. Because the fungus inhibits pigmentation, after treatment it takes time for the normal skin colour to return.

Abnormal pigmentation		
Disease	Colour and features	Surface
Vitiligo	White well-defined patches	Normal
Guttate hypomelanosis	White macules on arms	Normal
Melasma	Brown patches on face	Normal
Postinflammatory	Hyper- or hypopigmentation	Scaly
Pityriasis alba	Pale patches on cheeks	Scaly
Pityriasis versicolor	Uniform fawn/pink/brown	Slightly scaly
Fixed drug eruption	Red/brown patch/plaque	Scaly/vesicles/bullae
Morphoea	White/erythematous edge	Shiny indurated/ atrophic

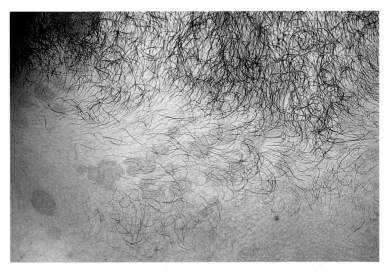

Fig. 34 Pityriasis versicolor.

Causes of papules, weals and nodules

Scabies

Scabies is becoming far more common. Certainly the GP should be highly suspicious when members of a family develop severe nocturnal itch. A papular rash is present on the axillary folds, around the umbilicus and on the thighs. Scabies is caused by infestation with a mite called *Sarcoptes scabiei*. The generalized itchy papular rash is caused by an immunological reaction to the mite. The classical lesions are burrows in the finger webs and on the sides of the hands; however, these are not always easy to find. In males it is worth examining the penis for papules. In babies and young infants the face, neck, soles and heels can be involved (Fig. 35).

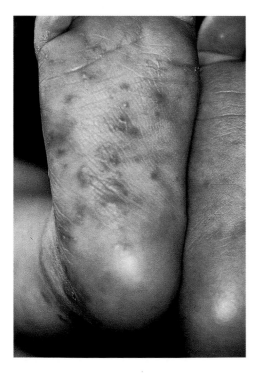

Fig. 35 Scabies—foot.

Causes of papules and nodules	
Disease	Features
Scabies	Very itchy with papules and burrows
Urticaria	Weals
Nodular prurigo	Multiple pink itchy nodules
Granulomatous sarcoid	Mauve papules without scale
Diffuse granuloma annulare	Erythematous papules without scale
Eruptive xanthoma	Multiple yellow papules
Neurofibromatosis	Café-au-lait patches and neurofibroma
Sweet's disease	Fever, tender plum-coloured lesions
Secondary melanoma deposits	Multiple pigmented nodules

Norwegian scabies

Patients with reduced immunity can become heavily infested with mites and a similar problem can arise in those who cannot scratch. The rash is rather psoriasiform in appearance and often goes undiagnosed. The patient then frequently infects other members of a nursing or residential home.

The itchy patient with a rash
- scabies—look for burrows and penile lesions
- urticaria—weals
- nodular prurigo—nodules and excoriations
- lichen planus—violaceous papules and oral involvement
- reaction to animal mites, similar to scabies

Dermographism

The skin reacts to pressure by becoming elevated and this can be tested for by writing with the blunt end of your pen on the patient's back. Dermographism appears quickly after pressure while pressure urticaria takes hours.

Acute urticaria

Acute urticaria presents as small and large weals. These are red raised itchy circumscribed areas of dermal oedema with no surface change (Fig. 36). It is not uncommon and lasts a couple of days. It is

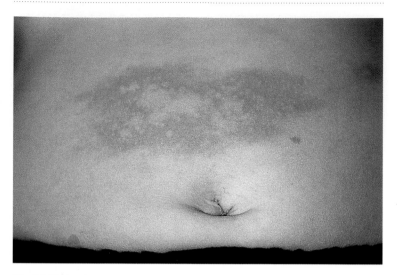

Fig. 36 Urticaria.

worth inquiring about any history of eating strawberries, taking penicillin or a viral infection.

Chronic urticaria

Chronic urticaria is that of at least 3 months' duration. For most cases there is no obvious cause. Some chronic urticaria may be associated with:

- salicylates
- azo dyes and benzoic acid preservatives in the diet
- myxoedema.

Although investigations are unlikely to give a positive result, in patients with chronic urticaria it is worth looking for treatable causes. Investigations for cases of chronic urticaria include:

- full blood count and erythrocyte sedimentation rate
- U&E, TFT
- MSU (mid-stream urine) and dipstick.

There are other types of urticaria, such as that produced by pressure and changes in temperature. If an individual weal of urticaria lasts more than 24h and there is bruising or arthralgia then one should consider a vasculitis.

Type of urticaria	Rash	Test
Dermographism	Immediate weal at the site	Scratch at site of pressure
Pressure	Delayed weal at site of pressure	Weights
Cholinergic	Multiple small weals	Heat and exercise
Cold	Weal at site of exposure	Apply an ice cube
Urticarial vasculitis	Weals >24 h leaving bruises	Immunological

Toxic erythema (Fig. 37)

An erythematous maculopapular rash resulting from a drug reaction or viral infection, e.g. penicillin allergy and measles.

Erythroderma

An ill patient presents with a confluent erythematous rash. There can be temperature regulation and fluid balance problems, therefore the patient needs urgent admission. The underlying pathology may not be obvious at this time; it may be eczema, psoriasis, drug reactions or lymphoma.

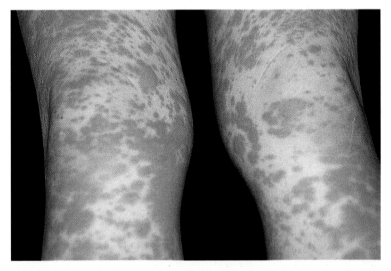

Fig. 37 Toxic erythema.

Granuloma annulare

This presents as an erythematous rash with a raised edge without scale. Lesions are classically found on the hands and feet although they can be widespread.

Erythema chronicum migrans

An annular erythema develops, possibly with the tick bite visible in the centre. This rash is associated with Lyme disease (Fig. 38), which results from infection with *Borrelia burgdorferi* via the tick.

Common blistering rashes

There are many causes of blistering rashes, some of which are very serious. However, usually when I am asked to give an opinion on a blistering eruption it is adults with chickenpox rather than pemphigoid or pemphigus.

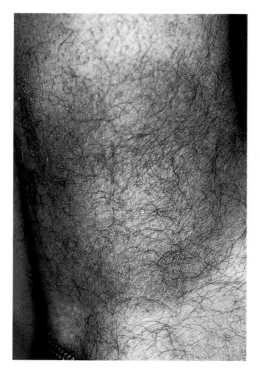

Fig. 38 Lyme disease.

Blistering with infection

Quite a few bacterial and viral infections can cause blistering. Bullae can occur with localized areas of impetigo, as the *Staphylococcus aureus* can release exotoxins. Staphylococcal infections in children can, in rare instances, produce a life-threatening scalded skin syndrome; there is a generalized erythema and shearing off of the skin to leave erosions. Adults develop an identical picture known as toxic epidermal necrolysis caused by a drug reaction. These patients need urgent hospital care for intensive treatment.

Blistering with infections	
Bacterial infection	Appearance
Impetigo	Flaccid bullae rupturing to leave yellow crusts
Chickenpox	Crops of papules and vesicles
Herpes zoster (Fig. 39)	Unilateral blisters following a dermatome

Rashes where blistering may be a feature

Some diseases can produce blisters in their more serious form. Most GPs are aware of the appearance the target lesions of erythema multiforme; however, there can also be blisters. Drug reactions

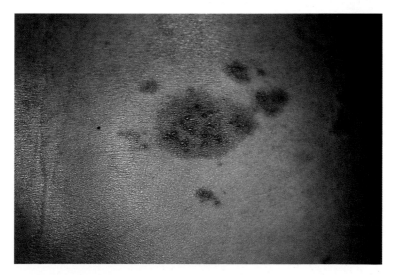

Fig. 39 Herpes zoster.

57

come in various guises. Most doctors have seen the classical wide-spread erythema of a penicillin reaction; however, only a few would recognize a blistering eruption caused by drugs.

Diseases where blistering may be a feature	
Disease	**Features**
Erythema multiforme	Multiple target lesions
Drug rashes	A wide spectrum
Contact allergic dermatitis (Fig. 40)	Bullae and erythema at site of contact
Phytophotodermatitis	e.g. plant juices interacting with sunlight, linear rash

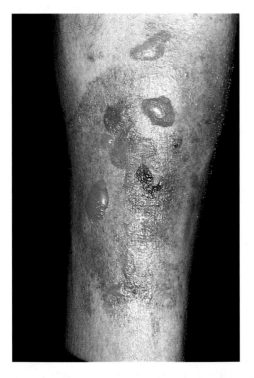

Fig. 40 Contact allergic dermatitis with blisters.

Inflammatory bullous diseases

The inflammatory bullous diseases are uncommon, but are serious and require early diagnosis. Therefore suspected cases should be referred to secondary care. Pemphigoid is more common than pemphigus and occurs in the elderly. Because the blister in pemphigoid is deeper in the skin it is less easily ruptured. The blister in pemphigus is more superficial and usually lost. Any rubbing of apparently normal skin causes loss of epidermis, this being known as Nikolsky's sign. Penicillamine and ACE inhibitors can produce drug-induced pemphigus.

Inflammatory bullous diseases	
Disease	Features
Pemphigus (rare)	Easily ruptured blisters leaving erosions, oral involvement and blisters on flexor surfaces of limbs
Pemphigoid	Intact tense blisters, localized or generalized affecting the extensor surfaces
Pemphigoid gestationis	Erythema and blisters during pregnancy
Dermatitis herpetiformis	Itchy patient with small blisters on buttocks, elbows and knees

Rashes on the lower legs

It is worth considering the lower leg in more detail as this is a common site of many rashes. When faced with a rash on the legs do palpate to see if it is hot, e.g. a cellulitis, or tender, e.g. erythema nodosum. In the summer insect bites are common on the lower limbs. Atopic eczema affects the popliteal fossae, psoriasis the knees and lichen planus the shins. Asteatotic eczema presents as dry scaly skin on the legs, with a rather crazy paving appearance (Fig. 41). Varicose eczema accompanies varicose veins, an eczematous eruption accompanied by oedema and pigmentation. The lower leg is a classical site for contact allergic dermatitis from dressings and topical antibiotics.

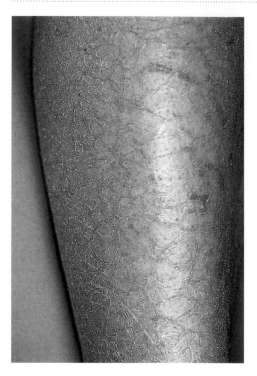

Fig. 41 Asteatotic eczema.

Rashes on the lower legs	
Disease	**Features**
Erythema nodosum	Tender red nodules on the pretibial areas
Necrobiosis lipoidica	Shiny yellow patches with red borders
Pretibial myxoedema	Nodules on the shins
Cellulitis	Hot swollen tender limb
Vasculitis	Painful palpable purpura
Weed whacker's dermatitis	Erythema with vesicles and bullae
Varicose eczema	Erythematous scaly rash with pigmentation
Asteatotic eczema	Dry scaly with crazy paving appearance
Contact allergic eczema	Eczema at site of creams or dressings
Bowen's disease	Pink scaly plaques

Erythema nodosum

Erythema nodosum appears as raised tender purple nodules on the extensor surfaces of the legs (Fig. 42). Erythema nodosum can be

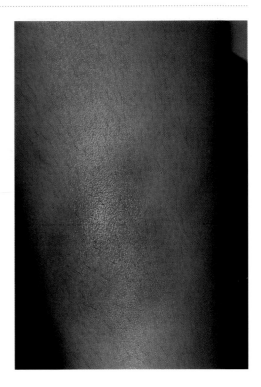

Fig. 42 Erythema
nodosum.

associated with streptococcal throat infections, sarcoid and drugs,
e.g. oral contraceptives and sulphonamides.

Necrobiosis lipoidica

Necrobiosis lipoidica presents as plaques on the shins, which have a
raised mauve edge and a yellow atrophic centre (Fig. 43). It is associated with diabetes mellitus.

Cellulitis of lower legs (Fig. 44)

There is a hot swollen limb with erythema. The patient can be unwell
with a fever and malaise. The infection of the subcutaneous tissues is
usually caused by streptococci which gain entry following tinea pedis
or a minor injury. Necrotizing fasciitis is caused by a streptococcal
infection, and the tabloids report cases as being caused by the 'flesh-
eating bug'. There is erythema, pain and tissue necrosis. The patient
is ill and needs urgent hospital attention.

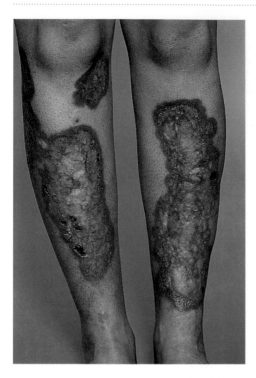

Fig. 43 Necrobiosis lipoidica.

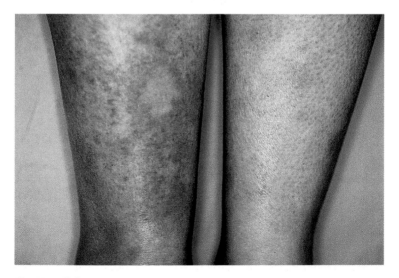

Fig. 44 Cellulitis.

Vasculitis

The presentations of a vasculitis can be quite diverse; however, lesions which do not blanch on pressure with a glass slide should stimulate one's interest. It can present as macules, papules and purpuric lesions. Henoch–Schönlein purpura presents in children and is often associated with a streptococcal sore throat. The purpuric macules and papules are found on lower limbs and buttocks.

Strimmer dermatitis (weed whacker's dermatitis)

Psoralen is contained in plants such as cow-parsley and cowslip. During strimming psoralen can be released onto the skin, to react with sunlight to produce a phytophotodermatitis. To aid diagnosis of rashes on the lower legs see Fig. 45.

Leg ulceration

Leg ulcers take up a lot of practice time and resources. Approximately 2% of a practice population has leg ulceration at some time in their lives and 80% of these cases will be venous in origin. One needs to aim to heal new ulcers quickly without side effects and avoiding undue expense.

Causes of leg ulceration:
- venous ulceration
- arterial ulcers
- diabetes mellitus
- rheumatoid arthritis
- malignancy
- pyoderma gangrenosum.

Chronic venous leg ulceration (Fig. 46)

Most leg ulcers will be venous in origin. Factors aiding diagnosis of venous insufficiency are that the ulcer affects the gaiter area and is relatively painless. There is venous hypertension with venous distension, dilated venules and a venous flare. There is often oedema, pigmentation and varicose eczema. The ulcer has an irregular, slightly raised edge and is accompanied by swelling and induration. If the foot pulses are not easily palpable, Doppler studies should be performed.

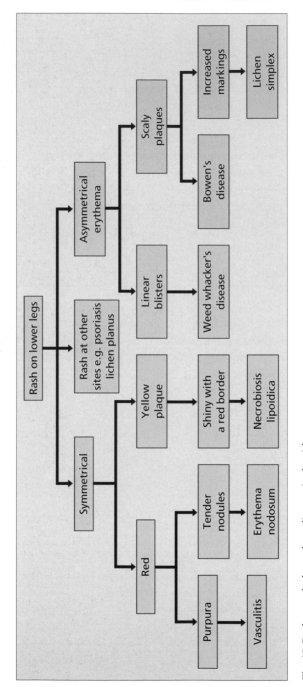

Fig. 45 Rashes on the lower legs: diagnostic algorithm.

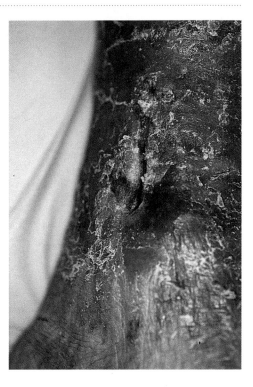

Fig. 46 Venous leg ulcer.

Ischaemic ulcer

It is very important that we know which ulcers are either arterial or have an arterial component (Fig. 47). This is to avoid cutting off the already compromised blood supply by compression bandaging. With ischaemia the ulcer is dry, painful and has a more punched out appearance. It can occur at any site. There may be a history of claudication and absent peripheral pulses. The skin is shiny and hairless with sluggish venous filling and poor capillary return. Ischaemic ulcers need the opinion of the vascular surgeon, and the practice must educate patients on the dangers of smoking and vascular disease.

General practice has a major role in the prevention of diabetic ulceration (Fig. 48). The diabetic foot needs special care with early intervention for any problem. Well-fitting shoes are a must. The practice team, and especially the diabetic clinic, have a key role in preventative care. Neoplastic change should be suspected if the ulcer

65

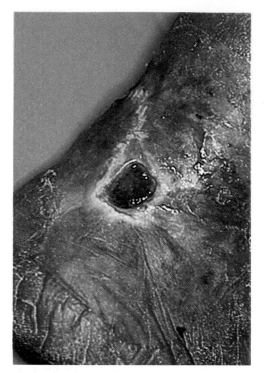

Fig. 47 Arterial ulcer.

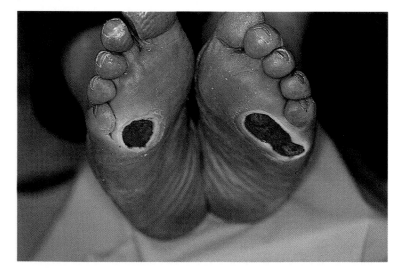

Fig. 48 Diabetic ulceration on the feet.

has a raised rolled edge or changes in size; a biopsy is then indicated. Pyoderma gangranosum can occur at any site. The rapidly growing ulcer has an overhanging edge and a violaceous colour.

Patients with special problems

Rashes in pregnancy

In pregnancy there is a changing hormonal status. Spider naevi appear and banal naevi tend to become darker which can cause some anxiety. The increasing girth results in stretch marks. There are some itchy conditions which can develop in pregnancy. Polymorphic eruption of pregnancy presents as a very itchy urticated rash with papules and vesicles; it is also known as pruritic urticarial papules and plaques of pregnancy. There is a much rarer and more serious condition of pemphigoid gestationis, in which there are not only similar lesions but also bullae.

Rashes in diabetes mellitus

Patients with diabetes are more prone to superficial skin infections. Patients with diabetes are more likely to have vitiligo. Necrobiosis lipoidica presents as shiny yellow patches on the shins with a red border. Only the diffuse form of granuloma annulare is associated with diabetes.

Autoimmune diseases

Certain dermatological conditions, e.g. alopecia areata and vitiligo, are associated with autoimmune disease. These diseases include pernicous anaemia, thyroid disorders and Addison's disease. Thyroid disease is associated with pretibial myxoedema.

Malignancy

One should always bear malignancy in mind when a patient presents with an undiagnosed itch. Various erythemas are associated with malignancy as is dermatomyositis. Velvety thickening in the flexures, acanthosis nigricans, is associated with malignancy.

Flexural rashes

Some diseases, such as erythrasma, only occur in the flexures; others, such as psoriasis, occur at many sites. However, the appearance is modified by being in a flexural environment. The flexures have their own microclimate; two surfaces come into contact which results in friction and increased hydration. Rashes in the flexures therefore have a paucity of scale and are frequently secondarily infected.

Differential diagnosis of flexural rashes	
Rash	Characteristics
Intertrigo	Moist, glazed red rash with secondary candidal infection
Tinea	Raised scaly edge with central clearing
Erythrasma	Uniform colour with no raised edge
Atopic eczema	History of atopy and rash at usual sites
Seborrhoeic eczema	Erythema and scaling with associated dandruff
Contact dermatitis	History of irritants or contact allergen
Lichen simplex	Lichenified, excoriated lesions with increased markings
Psoriasis	Well-defined edge, rash at other sites and nail deformity
Acanthosis nigricans	Pigmented velvety thickening of flexures with skin tags
Hidradenitis suppurativa	Abscesses, nodules and scars
Hailey–Hailey disease	Vesicles, fissures and crusts

Adapted with permission from *Exploring Eczema: a Distance Learning Package* (1995). Haymarket Publishing Services, London.

Flexural rashes

Intertrigo
This condition occurs in the flexures where there are two surfaces in contact producing a high humidity creating inflamed, oozing

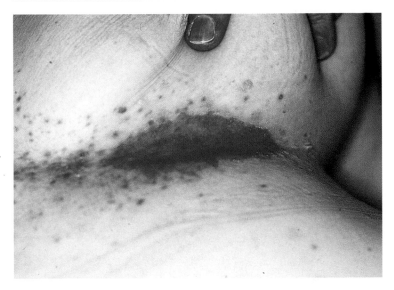

Fig. 49 Intertrigo.

and waterlogged skin (Fig. 49). The edge in intertrigo is less well-defined than in psoriasis and satellite pustules herald the presence of Candida.

Fungal infections
The flexures are common sites for fungal infections; dermatophyte and monilial infection may be primary or secondary to another dermatosis. The way not to miss a case is to take scrapings. It only takes a few minutes and it:
- enables one to confirm a diagnosis
- enables one to pick up atypical cases
- is always worth doing if a rash has not behaved as expected.

Dermatophyte infections
Tinea affects the male groin, it has a raised edge to the rash with scrotal sparing (Fig. 50). A search should be made for any evidence of tinea pedis and/or onychomycosis.

Erythrasma
Erythrasma occurs at flexural sites including the perineum and between the toes. It can also cause pruritus ani. The rash has a rather

69

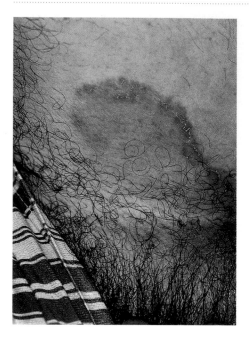

Fig. 50 Tinea cruris.

uniform colour with an even erythema. There is minimum scale and it does not have a raised edge in contrast to tinea. A Wood's light is useful and makes screening for this disease easy. The causative organisms are diphtheroids which produce porphyrins. Therefore there is coral-pink fluorescence.

Eczema

One should also ask about any atopic condition, such as asthma, eczema and hay fever. There may be signs at other sites which point to eczema as the diagnosis. With atopic eczema the cubital and popliteal fossae are involved and there is a generally dry skin. Clues to the diagnosis of seborrhoeic eczema might be a scaly scalp with a rash on the face in the nasolabial folds and behind the ears. A history of a new cosmetic or the finding of an unusual shape to the rash would suggest a possible contact allergic eczema.

Lichen simplex

Lichen simplex presents as a thickened lesion. This lichenification can be associated with excoriations and accentuated surface markings.

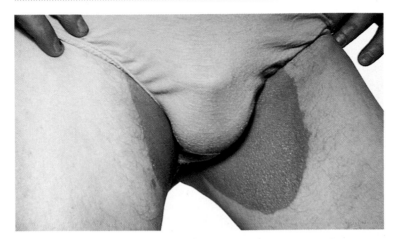

Fig. 51 Psoriasis in the flexures.

Psoriasis
Psoriasis in the flexures loses its silvery scale but retains its well-defined border (Fig. 51).

Hidradenitis suppurativa (Fig. 52)
Abscesses, nodules and scars form and one can think of this as acne of the flexures.

Acanthosis nigricans
The presence of a pigmented velvety thickening of flexures with skin tags is associated with malignancy (Fig. 53). A similar finding is found in the obese and those with diabetes mellitus.

Specific problems

Nappy rash
Nappy rash is a very common problem and is really a form of irritant eczema. The child presents with an erythematous rash in the napkin area, with sparing of the flexures. The rash occurs under the nappy in this warm moist area, subjected to the irritant effects of urine and faeces. Secondary fungal and bacterial infections are not uncommon. These result in the rash extending into the flexures and developing satellite pustules.

71

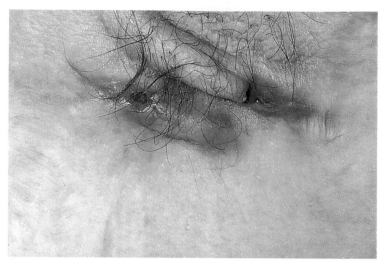

Fig. 52 Hidradenitis suppurativa.

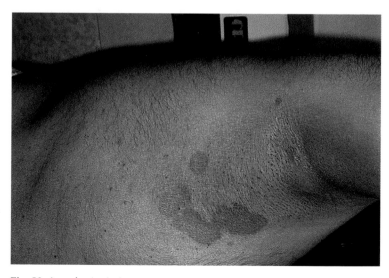

Fig. 53 Acanthosis nigricans.

Pruritus ani

Pruritus ani is common in overweight stressed males and has unkindly been labelled executive bottom by some. Many of the common dermatoses can affect the perineum. These include psoriasis, seborrhoeic dermatitis and eczema. Other dermatological problems include tinea lichen simplex and, rarely, lichen planus.

It is important to inquire into hygiene and faecal soiling or discharge. Piles are a very common cause of anal itch. With an anal fissure there is painful defaecation. One should exclude colitis and neoplasms, and inquire about any change in bowel habit or rectal bleeding. Threadworms need exclusion; placing a small piece of double-sided sellotape near the anus at night can provide a diagnosis next day. Prescribed or over-the-counter preparations can aggravate or perpetuate pruritus ani. The local anaesthetics cincochaine, amethocaine and benzocaine can produce a contact dermatitis.

Rashes on the genitalia

The vulva is an area where gynaecology, dermatology and common sense overlap. Not all that produces a rash is dermatological, and not all that patients complain of is physical. Some females develop discomfort in the vulva without any demonstrable pathology. Other females develop an atrophic vulva after the menopause. There are a whole host of conditions which affect the vulva and patients who defy diagnosis should be referred to those with a special interest.

Vulval rashes	
Diagnosis	Features
Candida	Itchy erythematous rash with white discharge
Lichen simplex	Itchy rash with increased markings
Lichen sclerosus et atrophicus	Shiny areas with pink borders
Leukoplakia	Thickened white plaques

Candidiasis is common; however, a balanitis in an elderly male which does not respond to antifungals should be referred to exclude an intraepidermal neoplasia. Genital lesions include herpes simplex type 1 or 2. Penile papules are pathognomonic of scabies.

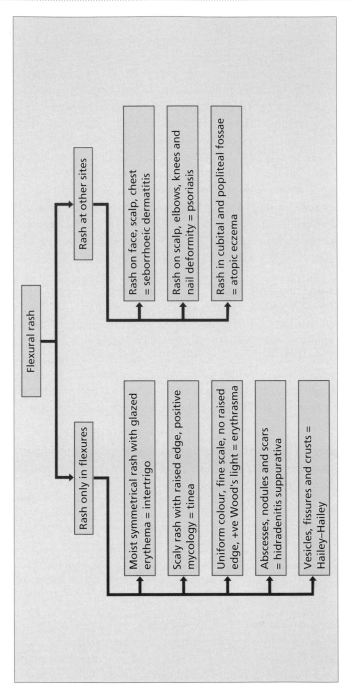

Fig. 54 Rashes in the flexures: diagnostic algorithm.

Flexural rash

Rash only in flexures

Rash at other sites

Moist symmetrical rash with glazed erythema = intertrigo

Scaly rash with raised edge, positive mycology = tinea

Uniform colour, fine scale, no raised edge, +ve Wood's light = erythrasma

Abscesses, nodules and scars = hidradenitis suppurativa

Vesicles, fissures and crusts = Hailey–Hailey

Rash on face, scalp, chest = seborrhoeic dermatitis

Rash on scalp, elbows, knees and nail deformity = psoriasis

Rash in cubital and popliteal fossae = atopic eczema

Penile rashes	
Disease	Appearance
Candidiasis	Erythema
Pearly penile papules	Small pearly papules on the corona
Psoriasis	Erythema with minimum scale and a rash at other sites
Lichen planus	Shiny flat-topped mauve papules
Scabies	Itchy red papules, rash at other sites
Genital warts	Pink/brown papules with warty surface
Herpes simplex	Erythema with vesicles

To aid diagnosis of rashes in the flexure see Fig. 54.

7 Hands and feet

The hands

The hands are capable of performing both heavy work and fine manipulation. They can act as a means of communication. As the hands are a visible site, rashes cause embarrassment. When faced with a rash on the hands one should observe:

• does it affect the hands and feet?
• does it affect the palms and soles?
• is it symmetrical?
• is it erythematous, are there vesicles, pustules or scale?

Common causes of symmetrical scaly red rashes on the hands and feet are psoriasis and endogenous eczema. A well-defined edge is present for plaque psoriasis, and pustules on the palms occur with localized psoriasis, while vesicles and blisters occur in pompholyx.

Rashes on the hands	
Disease	Characteristics
Plaque psoriasis	Red scaly rash with well-defined border
Pustular psoriasis	Yellow brown pustules on palms
Eczema (generic)	Erythema, lichenification and scaling
Pompholyx	Erythema and vesicles on the palms
Contact allergic eczema	Rash at sites of contact
Hyperkeratotic eczema	Erythema, hyperkeratosis and fissures
Scabies	Burrows between the fingers
Norwegian scabies	Thick fissured crusts
Knuckle pads	Found on young adults
Dermatomyositis	Violaceous plaques over knuckles
Tinea	Fine white scale on palms
Tinea on dorsum	Red scaly lesions with raised edge
Granuloma annulare (Fig. 55)	Raised red edge without scale

Hand eczema

Acute hand eczema has erythema, vesiculation and weeping. Secondary staphylococcal infection of eczema from any cause is

76

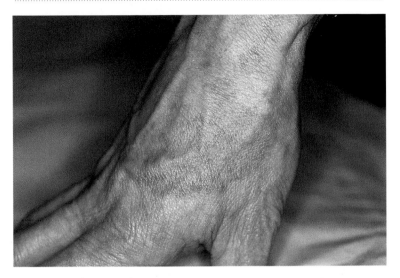

Fig. 55 Granuloma annulare.

common. Chronic eczema has scaling, lichenification and fissures on the digits. The cause of hand eczema is frequently multifactorial. One needs an occupational history and should also inquire into hobbies and pastimes. Patients such as hairdressers are very prone to hand eczema. Irritant hand eczema is more common than contact allergic dermatitis. Some substances, such as cement, can cause both an irritant and a contact allergic dermatitis. Bulbs can also produce both an irritant and allergic dermatitis on the fingers. Common causes of a contact allergic dermatitis are rubber gloves and chrysanthemums. The contact allergic dermatitis to the glove leaves a well-demarcated edge.

Factors to consider with an irritant dermatitis include:
• strength of irritant
• frequency of exposure
• individual susceptibility
• atopics are more susceptible.

Industrial hand dermatitis (Fig. 56)
This is a common problem and is often difficult to unravel. A high index of suspicion is required for those in at-risk occupations. One needs to inquire:

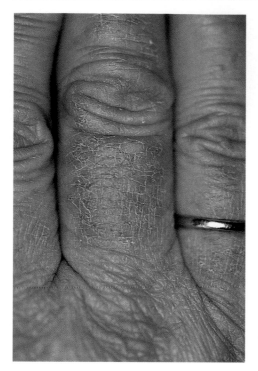

Fig. 56 Irritant contact dermatitis.

- how long the patient has been in their present occupation?
- what exactly does this involve?
- how long have they had the rash?
- does the rash improve on holidays?

Causes of irritant hand dermatitis	
Weak irritants	**Strong irritants**
Bulbs, e.g. onions	Cement
Detergents	Turpentine and white spirit
Soap	Trichlorethylene
Water and saline	Carbon tetrachloride
Weak acids	Petroleum and paraffin

Irritant induced dermatitis is more common than contact allergic dermatitis; however, most cases are multifactorial. Early referral for an opinion and patch testing is recommended. One has to remember not only the patient's occupation but also their hobbies. If a patient deteriorates rather than improves with treatment then a contact allergic reaction is a possibility.

Common allergens and where they are found	
Allergen	**Found**
Diallyldisulphides	Garlic
Chromate	Cement, leather and primer paint
Cobalt	Metal alloys and paint
Epoxy resins	Adhesives
Lactones	Chrysanthemums
Neomycin	Topical antibiotic
Paraphenylendiamine	Dye—clothing and hair
Preservatives, e.g. parabens and formaldehyde	Creams and cosmetics
Primin	The primula obconica
Rubber chemicals	Tyres, boots, gloves and shoes
Latex allergy (an immediate type of reaction)	Latex gloves

There can be what is known as an 'id reaction' to tinea on the feet, with a vesicular rash on the palms; this is produced by an immunological reaction to the tinea. Burrows between the fingers are pathognomonic of scabies.

When considering an asymmetrical rash one does need to know which is the dominant hand and which hand is used to perform certain tasks. There is the possibility of either a contact allergic dermatitis or a fungal infection. A contact allergic dermatitis has a well-demarcated edge. Tinea on the back of the hands presents as annular scaly areas with central clearing, while on the palms it appears as a fine scaly rash. Granuloma annulare is usually found on the dorsum of the hands and feet. It appears as annular red areas which have a raised edge and no surface change.

For those in farming communities orf is a common problem, it is caused by a pox virus which is endemic in sheep and is transmitted to farm workers. A papule forms at the site of contact on the hand, which goes on to become a painful pustule. There is no effective therapy, but orf does resolve spontaneously. Common and plane warts are found on the hands and verrucae on the feet. Candida can affect the proximal nail-fold in a chronic paronychia. It can also affect the web spaces between the fingers. Nail-fold telangiectasia are found in the collagen diseases.

The hands are exposed to sunlight, hence they suffer from solar damage and can develop light-related eruptions. Lentigines on the back of hands develop with sun exposure and are easily diagnosed as they are uniform in colour. Actinic keratoses present as rough scaly lesions.

Blisters and vesicles on hands and feet	
Disease	Features
Trauma, e.g. friction	Localized to site of trauma
Pompholyx	Blisters on palms and soles
Pustular psoriasis (Fig. 57)	Yellow brown pustules on hands and feet
Tinea	Itchy scaly rash on feet
Hand-foot-and-mouth disease	Lesions on hands and feet, ulcers in mouth
Orf	Blisters with possible haemorrhage and ulceration
Porphyria cutanea tarda	Blisters and scars on the dorsum of hands

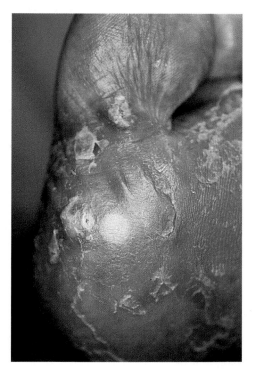

Fig. 57 Localized pustular psoriasis.

The feet

The prevalence of tinea pedis increases where there is communal bathing. The patient has itchy feet with maceration and scaling between the toes (Fig. 58); the most common site is between the fourth and fifth toes. There can be blisters associated with tinea on the feet which is worth diagnosing as it can be treated. Any rash that is unilateral, asymmetrical or not responding as expected to treatment may be of fungal aetiology.

Rashes on the feet	
Disease	Characteristics
Tinea pedis	Rash on feet, with involvement between the toes
Juvenile plantar dermatosis	Shiny glazed feet
Pitted keratolysis	Pits on soles of sweaty feet
Allergic contact eczema	Symmetrical rash from footwear, sparing of the toes
Plaque psoriasis	Scaly red rash, well-defined edge on hands and feet
Localized pustular psoriasis	Sterile yellow pustules turning brown, hands and feet
Hyperhydrosis	Moist palms and soles
Larva migrans	Itchy eczematous tract on foot

Juvenile plantar dermatosis is a condition which may be linked to atopic eczema (Fig. 59). The patient has shiny feet but no maceration between the toes as in tinea pedis. Pitted keratolysis is often confused

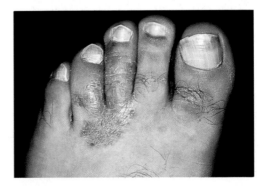

Fig. 58 Tinea pedis.

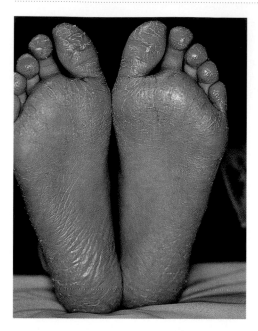

Fig. 59 Juvenile plantar dermatitis.

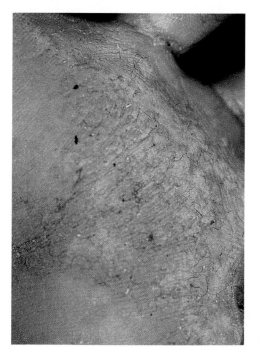

Fig. 60 Pitted keratolysis.

with tinea but once one has a mental picture of a classical case the problem is solved (Fig. 60); the patient having sweaty feet, multiple pits over the metatarsal heads and heels, but no scaling. Chromate in the leather of shoes can cause an allergic contact dermatitis, the demarcation of the rash following the outline of the leather.

Any acute eczematous process can produce blisters; however, they can also be a marker for viral infections. Hand-foot-and-mouth disease, as its name suggests, presents with vesicles on palms and soles together with mouth ulcers.

8 Abnormal nails

Nails are not just redundant appendages, they have a tactile and cosmetic value. When faced with a nail deformity one should consider:

- the type of nail deformity
- whether finger-nails and/or toe-nails involved
- whether multiple nails involved
- any concomitant rash
- taking mycological samples.

The most common nail deformities are those caused by fungal infections, psoriasis and trauma. Dermatophyte infections are usually of the toe-nails and Candida of the finger-nails. Dermatophyte infections produce thickened discoloured nails (Fig. 61). The deformity usually starts at the distal end of the nail and spreads proximally. This is in contrast to Candida, where the deformity starts proximally with a chronic paronychia.

The diagnosis of fungal nail infection is made by taking clippings for microscopy and culture. This needs to be carried out before a course of therapy is commenced. One should at least have positive microscopy. It can be impossible to differentiate fungal nail disease from psoriasis on clinical grounds.

Psoriasis can produce thickened nails with detachment of the nail from its bed, known as onycholysis (Fig. 62). Psoriasis also causes pits and salmon patches which help distinguish it from fungal nail disease. Pitting of nails can occur with both psoriasis and alopecia areata. Lichen planus can cause destruction of nails. It produces grooving and pitting of the nails. Lamellar splitting occurs in those who have their hands in water, the nails showing horizontal distal splitting. When eczema affects the pulps of the fingers it can cause a nail deformity.

A subungual haematoma as a result of trauma to the digit is common and one needs to exclude a melanoma. The haematoma does not involve the nail-fold. If there is any doubt one can scratch the proximal border of the discoloration of the nail and see it 'move down' the nail with time. If a white patient has a nail with a longitudinal pigmented streak involving the nail-fold, then melanoma needs

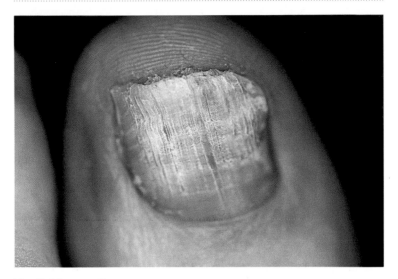

Fig. 61 Tinea—nails.

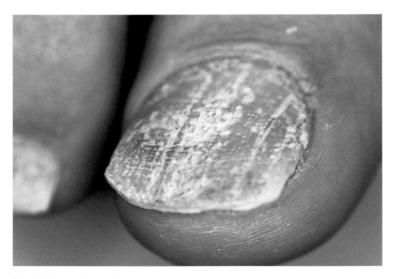

Fig. 62 Psoriasis—nails.

exclusion. Afro-Caribbean patients can present with streaks in multiple nails but these are not significant.

Causes and types of nail deformity	
Disease	Nail abnormality
Psoriasis	Thickening, onycholysis and pits
Dermatophyte	Thickening distal deformity with onycholysis
Candida	Paronychia affecting the nail-fold
Alopecia areata	Pits
Lichen planus	The cuticle grows down over nail-plate (a pterygium)

9 Lumps and bumps

So often in primary care patients ask 'While I'm here, doctor, could you just tell me what this is?' One can feel one's heart miss a beat as one hurriedly tries to decide that key question, is it benign or is it malignant? One can have a good stab at the diagnosis from:

- the age of patient
- the site of the lesion
- the appearance of the lesion
- single or multiple lesions
- the rate of growth of the lesion.

One can have a systematic approach, enquiring how long has a lesion been present, how quickly has it grown, and what brought it to the patient's attention.

Benign lesions

Viral warts

Warts are caused by the papilloma virus, and the appearance of the wart depends on the subtype of virus and the site of infection. Plane and filiform warts (Fig. 63) occur on the face. Plane warts often show Koebner's phenomenon, spreading along scars and excoriations (Fig. 64). Warts on the sole of the foot cannot grow outward because of the pressure and are therefore flat. Warts are usually multiple and have thrombosed capillaries within them which distinguishes them from callosities. Although warts commonly occur in childhood they can present at any age. However, one should take care if an elderly patient presents with a solitary 'warty lesion' not to miss a malignancy.

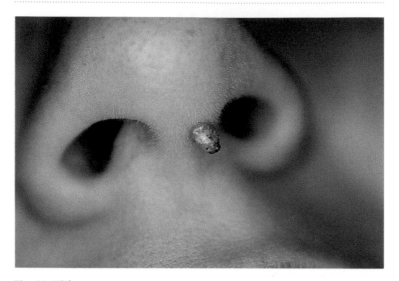

Fig. 63 Filiform warts.

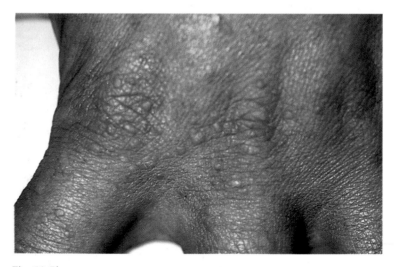

Fig. 64 Plane warts.

Warts		
Type	Site	Appearance
Common	Hands	Raised rough lesions
Filiform	Face and neck	Conical
Plane	Hands and face	Small slightly rough light brown papules
Verrucae	Soles of feet	Painful callous with black dots
Mosaic	Soles of feet	Coalescing verrucae

To differentiate a wart from a callosity:
- look for the thrombosed capillaries associated with a wart
- apply gentle side pressure — this is painful with a wart but not with a callosity.

Molluscum contagiosum (Fig. 65)
These lesions are caused by a pox virus and present as pearly papules with central umbilication. They can be multiple and are more common in those with atopic eczema. The actual molluscum may have an area of eczema around it.

Basal cell papilloma (seborrhoeic wart)
Basal cell papillomas are common, becoming more prevalent with

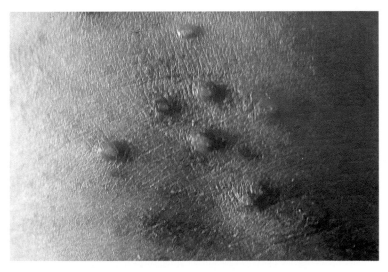

Fig. 65 Molluscum contagiosum.

increasing age and sun exposure. Despite sometimes being referred to as seborrhoeic warts they are not viral in aetiology. They are frequently found on the face and back. On the face they are only slightly raised, while on the back they have a rather stuck-on appearance and a cribriform surface. Sometimes one can see small keratin cysts on the surface, and it is worth picking at the lesions to aid diagnosis. Seborrhoeic warts have a uniform shape and colour which helps distinguish them from melanomas (Fig. 66). A seborrhoeic wart can become irritated, making exclusion of melanoma difficult. Applying a dressing for 2 weeks lets the architecture return to normal.

Dermatofibroma

Dermatofibromas are firm pigmented nodules which probably result from minor trauma. They are often found on the lower legs and may be itchy. Dermatofibromas dimple on squeezing because they are in the dermis and feel firm to touch.

Epidermoid cyst and pilar cyst

Cysts are found on the scalp and trunk. These are either epidermoid cysts or pilar cysts derived from the outer root sheath of the hair

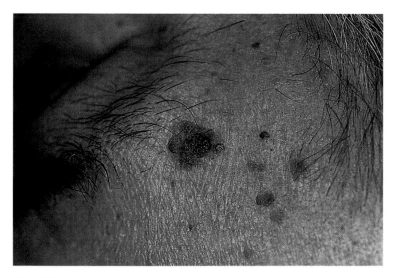

Fig. 66 Seborrhoeic warts.

follicle. It is possible to express cheesy material from epidermoid cysts. Tiny cysts that are found on the face are known as milia.

Keloids (Fig. 67)

Some patients are very prone to developing these firm nodules in scars. Afro-Caribbean patients often develop keloids in scars, therefore they should avoid ear piercing and their acne needs prompt attention.

Lipoma

Lipomas are benign tumours of fatty tissue, they are slow growing and have a soft rubbery feel.

Pyogenic granuloma

Pyogenic granulomas are red, very vascular rapidly growing benign lesions resulting from trauma. They are usually found on the fingers, but can occur on other sites. One needs to excise all lesions and send them for histology to exclude an amelanotic melanoma.

Chondrodermatitis nodularis chronica helicis

Very tender nodules develop on the ears of middle-aged or elderly patients which can be treated with cryotherapy or by surgery.

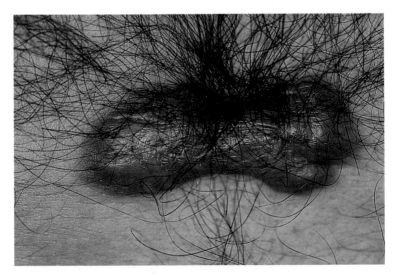

Fig. 67 Keloid.

Actinic keratosis (solar keratosis)

Actinic keratoses are hyperkeratotic erythematous scaly papules resulting from solar damage. The back of the hands and the bald scalp of elderly men are common sites. The lesions are easier to feel than see. Most actinic keratoses do not progress; however, a few may progress to become squamous cell carcinomas. Actinic keratoses can be treated with cryotherapy. However, if any lesion feels indurated and has substance then one needs to perform a biopsy to exclude a squamous cell carcinoma. All patients need advice on sun exposure, e.g. to wear a hat when gardening.

Cutaneous horn (Fig. 68)

The name is self explanatory although the diagnosis is not. A cutaneous horn needs excision and histology as it can be caused by:
• viral wart
• solar keratosis
• squamous cell carcinoma.

Keratoacanthoma

Keratoacanthoma is a fast-growing solitary lesion with a volcano-like centre found on a sun-exposed surface. Excision biopsy is required, as it can be quite difficult to distinguish the lesion clinically and histologically from a squamous cell carcinoma.

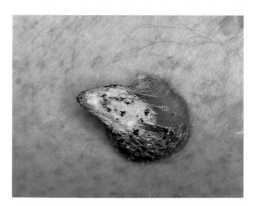

Fig. 68 Cutaneous horn.

Malignant lesions

Bowen's disease

This is a form of intraepidermal carcinoma, which can be related to solar damage and arsenic ingestion. Bowen's disease is commonly found on the lower legs, presenting as erythematous scaly plaques rather like psoriasis. It can be treated by cryotherapy, curettage or excision.

Basal cell carcinoma (Fig. 69)

Basal cell carcinomas commonly occur on the face and trunk of patients during middle and old age. They are often either cystic or nodular. They are pearly with telangiectasia and a rolled edge. The centre can break down leaving an ulcer covered by a crust. These features can be more obvious if one stretches the skin and picks off any crust. A basal cell carcinoma can also present as a non-itchy slowly enlarging plaque with a raised rolled edge. Some basal cell

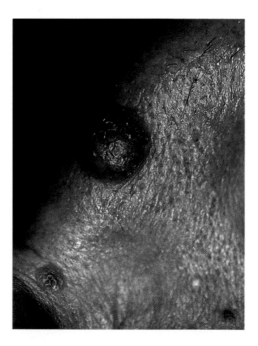

Fig. 69 Basal cell carcinoma.

93

carcinomas are pigmented. Methods of treatment include curettage, cryotherapy and excision biopsy.

Less common forms of basal cell carcinoma are:
- a scarring plaque known as a morphoeic basal cell carcinoma
- multicentric plaques of tumour.

Squamous cell carcinoma (Fig. 70)

Squamous cell carcinomas are less common than basal cell carcinomas. They occur at sites of solar damage, especially:
- the face, particularly the lower lip
- ears
- the bald scalp
- dorsum of hands.

Squamous cell carcinoma presents as an enlarging fleshy nodule on exposed surfaces such as on the face and hands. There can be a crust over the nodule which may ulcerate. The author remembers one elderly lady who had a small rather insignificant circular lesion at the angle of the mouth which turned out to be an squamous cell carcinoma.

Melanoma

Melanoma has sprung to the fore as attention has focused on this

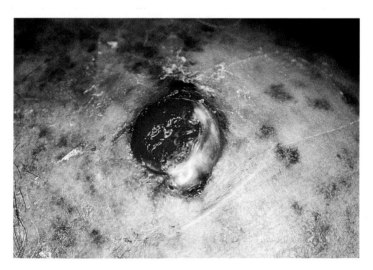

Fig. 70 Squamous cell carcinoma.

increasingly common malignancy which causes significant mortality to people at an early age. However, not all is doom and gloom as the prognosis for a patient with malignant melanoma depends on the thickness of the lesion at presentation. The early presentation and treatment of melanoma coupled with prevention by health education are the responsibilities of all members of the primary care team.

Risk factors for melanoma include:
• family history of melanoma
• fair hair, freckles and blue eyes
• presence of large congenital naevi
• presence of a large number of atypical naevi
• presence of multiple naevi
• short bursts of sunburn, especially in childhood.

Checklists aid in the diagnosis of melanoma; however, they are no substitute for clinical experience. The seven-point checklist for melanoma has a high sensitivity with specificity being of only secondary importance. If you can cover a naevus with the flat end of a pencil it is unlikely to be malignant.

Revised seven-point checklist for suspected malignant melanoma [9]	
Major signs	**Minor signs**
Change in size	Inflammation
Change in shape	Crusting or bleeding
Change in colour	Sensory changes
	Diameter = > 7mm

A patient with any one of the major signs should be considered for referral and the presence of any minor signs should be a further stimulus to referral. If you think a melanoma is likely then referral with full clinical information is probably most appropriate. If you think a melanoma is unlikely but there is some doubt one can either:
• perform an excision biopsy
• measure, record, photograph and review
• at review if still any doubt refer or perform excision biopsy.

The ABCDE checklist is commonly used in the USA [10].

ABCDE checklist
A Asymmetry
B irregular Border
C irregular Colour
D Diameter >6 mm
E Elevation

Palpating a pigmented lesion can aid diagnosis and is frequently overlooked. It is also worth measuring a pigmented lesion and recording your findings in the patient's notes. Photography can provide a useful record.

There are five types of melanoma:
- lentigo maligna
- superficial spreading
- nodular
- amelanocytic
- acral.

Lentigo maligna
Lentigo maligna is found on the faces of elderly patients. These macular lesions slowly increase in size, showing variation in pigment and having an irregular edge. They are now treated aggressively by surgical removal, as certain areas within the lesion can go on to develop a nodular phase.

Superficial spreading melanoma
This is the most common form of melanoma for young and middle-aged patients. It presents as a flat rapidly growing pigmented lesion which exhibits variation in pigment and asymmetry (Fig. 71). The most common presentation is of a rapidly changing pigmented lesion on the lower leg of a female patient.

Nodular melanoma
The melanoma can undergo vertical growth producing a nodular pigmented lesion (Fig. 72). These lesions account for approximately a quarter of melanomas. The most common site is on the patient's back.

Amelanotic melanoma
The melanoma can be without pigment and appear similar to a pyogenic granuloma.

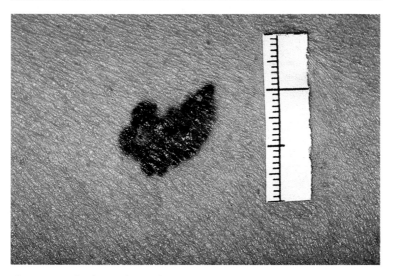

Fig. 71 Superficial spreading melanoma.

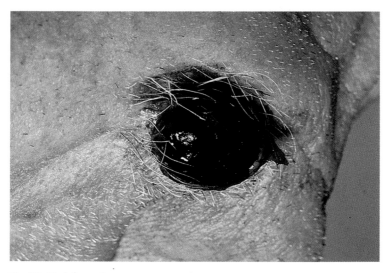

Fig. 72 Nodular melanoma.

Acral lentiginous melanoma
This is an aggressive nodular tumour on the palms and soles with a poor prognosis. These tumours are rare, but be suspicious of a new lesion around the first toe-nail.

10 Investigations, measurements and referrals

Investigations

Many specialities perform expensive, sophisticated and, at times, confusing investigations. Most dermatological investigations can be performed in primary care.

Bacterial investigations

Swabs sometimes confirm the clinical suspicions and on other occasions one is surprised. It can be difficult on clinical grounds to be sure if an infection is caused by either *Staphylococcus aureus* or *Streptococcus pyogenes*. Taking a swab:

- confirms the clinical diagnosis
- acts as a guide to appropriate antibiotics
- acts as a learning process.

Secondary bacterial infection is common with intertrigo and acute hand eczema, and it is worth taking a swab. With an acute paronychia one needs to take a swab to check that appropriate antibiotics are prescribed.

Mycological investigations

Taking mycological samples of skin, hair and nails is to be encouraged. Fungal infections are easily missed or incorrectly diagnosed. The frequent occurrence of tinea incognito highlights the need to be aware of the possibility of fungal infections and to take scrapings. Many fungal infections go untreated and substantial funds are wasted as a result of inappropriate prescribing of antifungals.

Samples can be taken of skin, hair and nails. They can be transported placed on black paper, using a commercial kit or making one's own, and can be sent or posted to a local laboratory or a mycological centre.

One needs to provide adequate samples of the affected material and provide full clinical details. Skin samples need to come from the active edge of the rash. The blunt outer edge of a stitch cutter blade can be used. From the scalp one can take scale and pluck affected hairs. A less traumatic alternative is to rub a disposable toothbrush over the affected area and then send it for culture.

When taking samples from nails one wants to send generous samples from the diseased area of the nail (Fig. 73). This is usually the distal nail with a dermatophyte infection and one can also include some of the debris from under the nail. Microscopy is available in days, culture can take 3 weeks. If mycology is negative and one is very suspicious of fungal nail disease then one should send more samples. If a patient has a superficial onychomycosis then one can take scrapings from the surface of the nail. If Candida is suspected, as with a chronic paronychia, then take a swab from the proximal nail-fold.

Viral swabs

Herpes simplex can be quite difficult to diagnose. It can present as a rash on the malar area or as a herpes whitlow. If there is any diagnostic difficulty it is worth taking a swab and sending it in viral transport medium to the local laboratory.

Wood's light

A Wood's light provides a quick non-invasive method of increasing

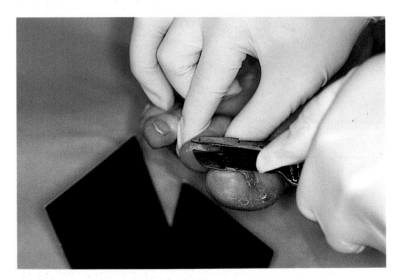

Fig. 73 Taking nail clippings.

one's diagnostic ability. There are some small hand-held battery operated models available which are inexpensive. The classical use of a Wood's light is in screening for tinea capitis. This can be to confirm one's clinical diagnosis or to screen asymptomatic contacts in a school. However, one needs to realize its limitations. Only certain species fluoresce; these include *Microsporum canis* and *Microsporum audouinii*. They produce green fluorescence. Screening can be performed on children in a school for contacts. Patches of pityriasis versicolor caused by the Pityrosporum yeast fluoresce yellow. Erythrasma is caused by a Corynebacterium which produce porphyrins that fluoresce green (Fig. 74). It is worth viewing patients with vitiligo under a Wood's light as this delineates patches which could have been clinically missed.

Patch testing
Patch testing is used to diagnose contact allergic dermatitis. This is

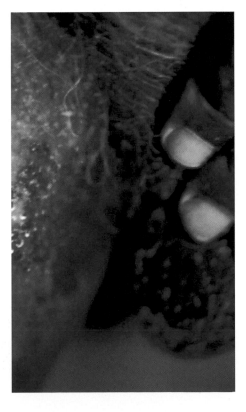

Fig. 74 Erythrasma under a Wood's light.

not uncommon, e.g. one in 10 females is allergic to nickel. This test works on delayed hypersensitivity. One applies probable and possible substances on patches on the patient's back and reads the result in 48–72h. There is a European standard battery, and then there are batteries to cover special problems, such as hairdressing and cosmetics. One can get false-positive and -negative results. Reactions produced by contact irritants can add to the confusion. One therefore needs expertise in performing and interpretation of patch tests, and they are not a routine screening test. Patch testing is important with industrial dermatitis; however, there are medicolegal connotations.

The repeated open application test is a simple procedure which one can perform in primary care. A small amount of the substance in question is placed on the elbow and one observes over the subsequent week for any reaction.

Prick test

Although used as a research tool, this test is of little value in daily practice. For latex allergy one would be advised to perform a blood test.

Blood tests

In dermatology in any case of unexplained itch it is worth checking the full blood count (FBC) and erythrocyte sedimentation rate (ESR) together with the urea and electrolytes (U&E), liver function tests and thyroid function tests. In cases of recurrent candidiasis it is worth performing a random blood sugar test to exclude diabetes.

Immunology

Because latex allergy is an immediate hypersensitivity reaction a blood test is the appropriate investigation, not a patch test. The FBC and ESR and immunological screen is useful in connective tissue disorders. Immunological tests include the ANF, DNA, Ro, La, ENA and cardiolipin antibodies. In cases of severe urticaria accompanied by anaphylaxis or obstruction of the airway, it is worth screening for hereditary angioedema, by asking for the C1 esterase inhibitor level and a C4 level.

Investigation of generalized pruritus	
Test	Reason
FBC and ESR	Anaemia, neoplasm
Ferritin	Anaemia
Thyroid function tests	Myxoedema
Creatinine and U&E	Renal failure
Liver function tests	Liver disease
Chest X-ray	Neoplasms

The Doppler ultrasound scanner (Fig. 75)

Compression bandaging may produce a disaster with irreversible tissue damage and possible amputation. More than 10% of venous ulcers can have an unrecognized arterial component. The only sure way to pick up these cases is with a Doppler scanner. With the hand-held Doppler scanner the ratio of ankle/brachial pressure is a guide

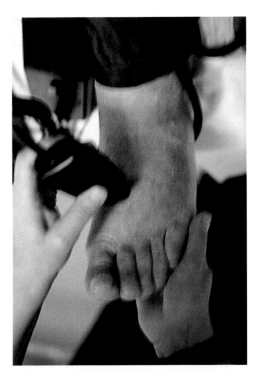

Fig. 75 Doppler scanning being performed.

to the severity of arterial disease. The ratio of systolic blood pressure at the ankle to that at the arm should be >0.8. This service can be provided by the practice nurses who have had appropriate training. Measurements are not reliable in those with diabetes mellitus.

Biopsy

The surgeon's maxim was 'when in doubt cut it out'. However, in dermatology if you do not know what a lesion is the pathologist may also have difficulty with the diagnosis and it would have been better to let the dermatologist see the lesion *in situ* first.

Guidelines for biopsying rashes

Biopsy of a rash is often unhelpful unless [11]
- there is a good differential diagnosis
- the correct biopsy site has been selected
- the result can be discussed with a dermatopathologist

Biopsy of rashes or tumours prior to referral to a dermatologist is unnecessary

---

Only do a biopsy if you have a working diagnosis: do not do it blindly. It is much better to do an excision, rather than an incisional biopsy of a lesion, as there is a theoretical risk of spread of melanoma. There has been concern that GPs are more likely to excise melanomas unknowingly than hospital doctors [12]. If one suspects a lesion is a melanoma then referral is probably the best action. However, if one thinks the lesion is probably benign but there is still an element of doubt it is worth doing an excision biopsy. Excision biopsy and histological assessment is the gold standard and certainly all atypical, changing or asymptomatic naevi should be excised [13].

Immunofluorescence

Immunofluorescence is used to distinguish different forms of blistering disorders and makes colourful slides for lectures! The direct method uses a biopsy of the patient's skin. Characteristic patterns are:
- IgA near the basement membrane in dermatitis herpetiformis
- IgG within the epidermis in pemphigus vulgaris
- IgG antibodies at the basement membrane in pemphigoid.

Indirect immunofluorescence detects antibodies in the patient's serum. This test can be useful in pemphigus and pemphigoid.

Photography of moles

Clinical diagnostic accuracy may be enhanced by offering clinicians managing suspicious melanocytic skin lesions a simple algorithm and a camera with which to record the appearance of lesions objectively [14]. A photograph can be sent together with a referral letter to convey the appearance of the rash or lesion at the time of referral.

Measurement in dermatology

A simple ruler enables pigmented lesions to be measured and the result recorded in the notes. A patient's skin type can be assessed by inquiring into their ability to tan or tendency to burn with sunshine. However, it may be easier in practice just to record, for example, a fair-skinned redhead.

Skin type	Characteristics
I	Always burn, never tans
II	Sometimes burn, rarely tans
III	Rarely burn, tans easily
IV	Never burn, always tans
V	Asian subjects
VI	Afro-Caribbean

There are various measurements of the clinical severity of skin diseases:
- acne — comparison with standard grading pictures;
- eczema — the SASSAD [15]; and
- psoriasis — the psoriasis area severity index score (PASI).

However, the effect on quality of life is generally more important than the actual extent of a rash.

Quality of life measurement

Skin disease affects patients in many different ways. There is the loss of function associated with such problems as a hand eczema or a nail dystrophy. The persistent scaling of a rash, such as psoriasis, can result in problems with clothing, bedding and bathing. A disease such as acne can flare in a tropical climate and exclude a patient from joining the armed services. Rashes can cause patients embarrassment and can result in prejudice. Patients with acne are less likely to find employment.

The effect of a rash is not simply related to its extent. Rashes which affect visible sites or affect the performance of daily tasks are more likely to have an effect on quality of life. The inflammatory dermatoses cause most problems.

One can use a general health questionnaire such as the SF-36; however, these are not very disease-specific for dermatology [16]. A general dermatological questionnaire is of more value and can be used to compare the impact of different skin diseases [17]. The dermatology life quality index (DLQI) was designed for practical use in a clinical setting to aid clinical decision-taking, audit and clinical research [18]. Research using the DLQI has shown that there is a high impairment of the quality of life of adults with skin disease in primary care [19]. Disease-specific questionnaires, such as those for acne and psoriasis, are quite sensitive but obviously do not enable comparisons between diseases to be made [20, 21]. One can devise a questionnaire looking at the problem from the family's perspective [22].

Questionnaires for measuring the impact of skin disease include:
• general health (SF-36)
• adults with skin disease (DLQI)
• children with skin disease (CDLQI)
• acne (CADI and APSEA)
• psoriasis (PDI).

Referrals

Secondary care should complement primary care and not be a substitute for it. Referrals should be of benefit to the patient and also carry an educational component to all concerned. It is worth stating what the patient and GP hope to gain from the referral and secondary care should try to address these issues. We have seen the development of specialized clinics, such as the pigmented lesion clinic, designed to cope with the increasing prevalence of skin cancer. One can help secondary care by providing full details.

Suggested contents of referral letter for melanoma:
• what features prompted referral, e.g. change in size, shape or colour

- over what timescale the changes have occurred
- risk factor, e.g. family history of melanoma, multiple atypical naevi, fair hair, etc.
- whether melanoma is truly suspected
- patient's degree of concern and knowledge.

It has been suggested that GPs could make more appropriate use of pigmented lesion clinics, and clinics should send GPs an annual reminder about the service and its purpose [23].

Increasingly, patients are referred to an open access clinic just for a test, e.g. patch testing. While this can be beneficial, results need careful interpretation. Advances in technology are enabling the diagnosis to be made far from the 'bedside' and this will continue as video images improve. High-resolution digital cameras can be used in conjunction with laptop computers to enable good quality pictures to be sent electronically. Teledermatology has the potential to be of benefit to physicians and patients, but it should not de-skill those in primary care.

The referral letter should outline the natural history of the patient's condition. In dermatology, family history and occupational history are often important. If the referral is marked urgent then it is best to state why, expanding on the degree of concern of either the doctor or patient. It is very helpful to know what problems the rash causes for the patient and how motivated he or she is regarding treatment.

A printout of the practice computer's information on a patient can be useful. This is especially helpful in trying to unravel what treatment he or she has had, and for what duration. This stops patients leaving the dermatology department with the same ineffective medication they had been given previously. It also enables one to make sure that patients have had an adequate dosage and duration of treatment, e.g. oral antibiotics for acne.

If preliminary investigations are performed in primary care this can speed the decision-making at consultation in secondary care:
- screening of lipids, LFTs and blood sugar before oral retinoids
- ferritin and thyroid function in diffuse alopecia
- serum testosterone level in cases of hirsutism
- mycological samples from a nail dystrophy.

Now it is time to go on and treat some patients!

11 Managing common skin diseases

Most patients want to know more about their skin problem. Often they just want reassurance that their rash is not infectious, or that their tumour is not malignant. Different patients react differently to a rash of equal severity. Certainly one needs to know what psychological problems a rash creates, and how it affects daily living. Factors affecting treatment include:

- the site and severity of the rash
- the efficacy of therapy
- the cosmetic acceptability of treatment
- the time involved in daily treatment
- the duration of treatment.

A patient's goals from treatment might be quite different from that of their physician, e.g. if they have psoriasis they may just want short-term therapy for a major forthcoming event, such as a marriage. The speed of improvement with therapy is important; patients soon become disillusioned with therapy if this is not rapid. Patients need an explanation of how long treatment will be needed, and how soon they are likely to relapse on cessation, if ever. Patients do not continue with therapy if there are major side effects. The most common skin diseases and therapies are discussed in detail in the following chapters, while other conditions and therapies are included in note form.

Management of acne and other facial rashes

Treating facial rashes

The face is a very important visible site, where therapies must be cosmetically acceptable. One should use a formulation which spreads easily and is not greasy, e.g. a cream or lotion. Many therapies which can be used on the trunk and limbs may irritate when applied to the face and flexures. These include dithranol and vitamin D analogues. One should avoid using potent topical steroids on the face and flexures because of the increased risk of side effects. Discoid lupus erythematosus is an exception to this rule, as it produces such profound scarring. One would be well advised not to attempt to alter facial pigmentation unless one has expertise in this field.

Acne

At puberty there is a physiological increase in androgen production and some patients have sebaceous glands which are more sensitive to these physiological levels of androgens. Factors involved in the aetiology of acne and which one can try to reverse with therapy are:
- increased sebum excretion
- obstruction of the pilosebaceous duct
- colonization with the anaerobe *Propionibacterium acnes*
- production of inflammation.

The overriding objective is to improve the patient's appearance and prevent scarring. One needs to find a therapy which is acceptable to each patient. Topical therapies are appropriate for mild to moderate acne, while more severe acne requires the introduction of an oral therapy. Certain sites, such as the patient's back, are difficult to treat with a topical therapy.

The treatment of acne depends on:
- the predominant type of lesion
- the sites involved

- the severity of the condition
- the patient's wishes.

Topical therapy for acne

When deciding which topical therapy is most appropriate, one needs to know whether comedones or inflammatory lesions predominate. Benzoyl peroxide is the gold standard of topical treatments for acne. It treats both inflamed lesions and comedones. Benzoyl peroxide does produce irritation and can cause bleaching of hair and clothing. The irritation can be overcome by gradually increasing the potency of benzoyl peroxide and by using emollients. The initial application of benzoyl peroxide should be for only 15 min and the time is gradually increased with subsequent applications. An alternative to benzoyl peroxide is azelaic acid. This is less irritant, more expensive and occasionally can cause photosensitivity. It can be helpful in cases of hyperpigmentation. Topical nicotinamide is another topical therapy which acts by reducing inflammation rather than acting against the *P. acnes*.

Topical antibiotics

Topical antibiotics are a cosmetically acceptable way of treating inflamed acne lesions. Frequently prescribed preparations include clindamycin and erythromycin. Although topical antibiotics overcome the systemic side effects of oral antibiotics, they can predispose to the development of bacterial resistance. Combining topical erythromycin with either benzoyl peroxide or zinc reduces the development of bacterial resistance.

To reduce bacterial resistance one should:

- not use concomitant different oral and topical antibiotics
- use the same effective antibiotic for a particular patient for repeated courses
- not continue with antibiotics longer than necessary.

Topical retinoids

Topical retinoids are very useful where comedones predominate. Irritation can occur with topical retinoids, especially during initial therapy. Photosensitivity can be another problem; however, restricting treatment to evening applications can overcome this side effect. A topical retinoid antibiotic combination is useful for patients who do not want to take an oral therapy.

Topical treatment of acne		
Topical	Advantage	Disadvantage
Benzoyl peroxide	Gold standard, but rather utilitarian	Irritation
Azelaic acid	Less irritation than benzoyl peroxide	Cost
Antibiotics	Acceptable, ideal for inflammatory lesions	Bacterial resistance
Retinoids	Effective against comedones	Irritation
Combinations	More effective and less bacterial resistance	As individual drug

Oral antibiotics

Oral antibiotics are the mainstay of the treatment of moderate acne. They are given in combination with a topical agent, usually benzoyl peroxide. Tetracycline is usually given in a dosage of 500 mg twice daily half an hour before food. This drug needs to be given for 6 months, although the dosage can be reduced at 3 months if there are side effects. The usual problem is a gastrointestinal upset. If there is no improvement in the acne at 3 months then bacterial resistance may be the problem and it is advisable to change antibiotic. It may be worth patients having a two-week antibiotic holiday during prolonged courses of antibiotic as this may help reduce the level of resistant *P. acnes*. The patient should continue with topical benzoyl peroxide during this 'wash out' period.

Tetracyclines should not be given to children under 12 years of age or to females during pregnancy, as tetracycline can stain developing teeth and may be taken up by bone. Erythromycin does not cause these problems, therefore some physicians would use erythromycin as a first-line therapy for female patients; however, resistance to this drug is becoming a real problem. Erythromycin should be given in the same dosage as tetracycline. Oral antibiotics can transiently interfere with absorption of the combined oral contraceptive pill; therefore extra precautions should be taken for some weeks when oral antibiotics are introduced.

Minocycline is a useful second-line antibiotic therapy for acne, as there is a low level of bacterial resistance and it can be given once daily. A rare side effect of minocycline is pigmentation (Fig. 76). Minocycline also has some even rarer but more serious side effects; these include an eosinophilic pneumonitis and a lupus-like

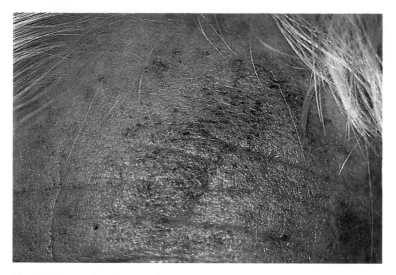

Fig. 76 Minocycline pigmentation.

syndrome, which is reversible on cessation of minocycline. Minocycline has been associated with an autoimmune hepatitis [24]. Some workers have suggested that tetracycline or oxytetracycline should be the first-line treatment of acne [25]. Doxycycline has the advantage of a once daily dosage regime; however, photosensitivity can be a problem. Trimethoprim is a promising drug for the future treatment of acne which GPs are used to prescribing for urological problems.

Oral antibiotics for acne

Drug	Dosage	Benefit	Major concern
Tetracycline	500 mg b.d.	Inexpensive	Gastrointestinal upset
Erythromycin	500 mg b.d.	Use in pregnancy	Bacterial resistance
Minocycline	100 mg o.d.	Low resistance	Pigmentation and serious rare side effects
Doxycycline	50 mg o.d.	Once daily	Photosensitivity
Lymecycline	408 mg o.d.	Once daily	As tetracycline
Trimethoprim	Variable	Difficult cases	No product licence, rashes

Hormonal therapy

Cyproterone acetate is an antiandrogen. It is combined with ethinyl-oestradiol in a propriety product, Dianette, a medication that is both a contraceptive and an acne therapy for the female patient. It has the same contraindications as a combined oral contraceptive. Dianette also has some beneficial effects for women with hirsutism. Patients taking Dianette should receive concomitant topical therapy, e.g. benzoyl peroxide.

Indications for oral retinoids

Oral retinoids are indicated for severe nodular acne and for those cases of severe acne which have not responded to adequate anti-biotic therapy. It is vital to prevent scarring as this is very difficult to treat. The risk of suicide with dermatological conditions has been highlighted. One study reported 16 deaths from patients who had presented to two dermatologists. There were seven men and nine women and most patients had either a body image dis-order (dysmorphophobia) or acne [26]. Oral retinoid therapy can help patients with psychological problems related to their acne; however, there is a slight risk of depression associated with this medication.

Oral isotretinoin

- Indications include severe nodulocystic and severe acne not responding to therapy.
- Oral isotretinoin is highly teratogenic.
- Contraception—during and for one month after cessation of isotretinoin.
- Side effects—hair loss, nose bleeds, sore lips and dryness of mucous membranes.
- Biochemical problems—can elevate lipids.

Patients on retinoids need to be advised of the probable local side effects such as sore lips and nose. Oral retinoids are highly teratogenic, therefore female patients must not become pregnant during treatment and for one month after cessation of therapy. They must have adequate contraception and receive appropriate advice.

When choosing a treatment for acne, the following algorithm may be useful (Fig. 77).

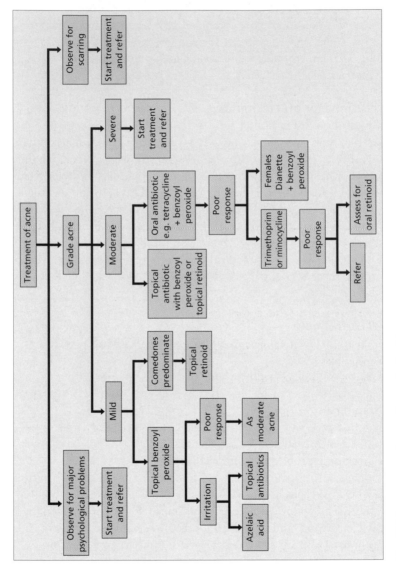

Fig. 77 The treatment of acne: diagnostic algorithm.

Indications for referral of cases of acne:
- severe nodulocystic acne
- patients not responding to adequate first-line therapy
- any evidence of a tendency to scarring
- hyperpigmentation

Other facial rashes

Rosacea
The treatment of rosacea is similar to that of acne; however, there are no comedones to treat. A 6–12-week course of tetracycline or erythromycin is usually effective at reducing the inflammatory lesions of papules and pustules. The erythema is very difficult to treat and one can try symptomatic remedies, e.g. emollients. Green cream can be applied to reduce the visible erythema. Aggravating factors for patients with rosacea include:
- hot drinks
- alcohol
- spices
- excessive heat and sunshine.

Diseases covered in other sections
- Psoriasis (see p. 127).
- Seborrhoeic eczema (see p. 122).

Perioral dermatitis
- Gradual withdrawal of any topical steroids being applied.
- Oral tetracycline or erythromycin.
- Emollients.

Sycosis barbae
- Oral flucloxacillin.
- Oral erythromycin.
- Topical antiseptics.

Chloasma/melasma
- Check for causative and/or aggravating medications, e.g. the contraceptive pill.

- Advice on sun exposure.
- Possible role for azelaic acid.

Discoid lupus erythematosus
- Usually under secondary care.
- Can affect other sites.
- Potent topical steroids.
- Sunscreens.
- Antimalarials.

Antimalarials
- Indications for hydroxychloroquine—systemic and discoid lupus erythematosus.
- Hydroxychloroquine—regular ophthalmic checks as risk of retinopathy.
- Indication for dapsone—dermatitis herpetiformis.
- Dapsone—monitor FBC, risk of haemolytic anaemia.

Treatment of solar-related conditions

Sunlight can provoke attacks of herpes simplex and aggravate conditions such as Darier's disease and porphyria. Most patients with psoriasis improve with sunlight but a few are aggravated by it.

Polymorphic light eruption
- Sunscreens—high factor against UVA.
- Topical steroids.
- Oral sedative antihistamines.

Solar urticaria
- Sun avoidance.
- Sunscreens.
- Oral non-sedative antihistamines.

Treatment of solar reactions
- Analgesia.
- Sun avoidance.
- Topical steroids short-term.
- Calamine lotion.
- Look for drug-induced phototoxicity/photoallergy.

Management of eczema

The treatment of eczema

The aetiology, and indeed the treatment, of many of the different types of eczema overlap. Most cases of eczema need a topical steroid in the short- to medium-term, to bring the rash under control. In the long term the GP should encourage the use of emollients, bath emollients and soap substitutes. Obviously it is desirable to exclude any aggravating or causative factors. When eczema is acute one wishes to increase the potency of the topical steroid and use a cream formulation. In the long-term one requires the weakest steroid possible in an ointment formulation.

Which topical steroid to use on different types of eczema

Type of eczema	Acute	Chronic
Infantile atopic eczema	Weak or moderate steroid	Weak steroid
Adult atopic eczema	Potent steroid	Weak or moderate steroid
Any facial eczema	Weak steroid	Weak steroid
Flexural eczema	Weak steroid and antimicrobial	Weak steroid
Seborrhoeic eczema	Weak steroid and antimicrobial	Weak steroid and antifungal
Hand and foot eczema	Potent steroid	Moderate potency steroid
Discoid eczema	Potent steroid and antibiotic	Moderate potency steroid
Stasis eczema	Weak or moderate steroid	Weak steroid

Adapted with permission from *Action Plans for Ezcema Management: A Report from a Workshop on the Management of Eczema in General Practice: May 1994*: Update 4, 1998; p. 432. Colwood House Medical Publications, Reading.

Eczema and infection

It is worth taking a swab if eczema deteriorates, as secondary bacterial infection and/or colonization is common. The usual pathogen is *Staphylococcus aureus* although it can occasionally be a *Streptococcus pyogenes*. Bacterial infection can have a direct irritant effect on the skin. Superantigens are produced by certain strains of *S. aureus* which colonize eczema, and these superantigens can have a deleterious effect on the eczema [27]. It is therefore worth considering antibiotics in the short term, and antiseptics in the long term when treating eczema. In an acute flare of eczema one can:

- initiate a topical steroid or increase its potency
- prescribe a course of oral flucloxacillin or erythromycin
- prescribe a combined topical steroid and antibiotic, e.g. fusidic acid with hydrocortisone or betamethasone valerate.

If a patient has recurrently infected eczema it might be because they or their families are nasal carriers of *S. aureus*. This can be reduced by using a course of mupirocin nasal ointment. The Pityrosporum yeast plays some part in seborrhoeic eczema, and topical antifungals have a beneficial therapeutic effect. One can prescribe ketoconazole cream and shampoo.

Herpes simplex infection on atopic skin can produce a very florid rash with a very toxic patient; a condition known as eczema herpeticum. A patient who has eczema and develops herpes simplex needs urgent treatment with systemic antivirals. Patients with atopic eczema should avoid close contact with people with active cold sores. Infection with the chickenpox virus can produce similar results, and children who have atopic eczema and develop chickenpox should be treated early with oral aciclovir.

Atopic eczema

Parents who have a child with atopic eczema want to do everything they can for their child. The outlook for children with atopic eczema is generally quite good, although one cannot promise this in individual cases. The rash can also recur in later life, especially if the skin is exposed to insults by the choice of an inappropriate occupation.

The treatment of atopic eczema includes:

- topical steroids

- emollients
- bath emollients and soap substitutes
- beating the itch–scratch cycle
- countering the hostile environment.

Bathing and eczema

Patients with atopic eczema need to take care of their skin. Bathing reduces the bacterial colonization; however, soap has an irritant effect. Patients should have a warm rather than a hot bath and should avoid soap by using a soap substitute. The skin should not be scrubbed and patients should use a bath emollient. The skin should be patted dry rather than vigorously rubbed. If the patient wishes to apply a steroid this should be done straight after the bath when there is maximum skin hydration, or 20 min after the application of an emollient. Holidays and modest sun exposure are beneficial; however, one needs to avoid increasing the risk of melanoma from excessive or intense exposure. After swimming the patient should shower to remove irritants, e.g. chlorine.

Beating the eczema itch–scratch cycle

It is very important to take appropriate measures to break the itch–scratch cycle. Finger-nails should be short to reduce the damage from scratching. It is important not to give purely negative messages. Suggest patting the skin as an alternative to scratching. The patient should wear either cotton clothing or a material with a high cotton content to reduce irritation. Non-biological washing powders are to be encouraged. Short courses of sedative antihistamines can be beneficial in reducing the itch. Wet wraps using a stockinet suit or occlusive bandages can be helpful (Fig. 78).

Massage has been advocated as a therapy for atopic eczema. Certainly it should help overcome a feeling that atopic eczema is unattractive and/or untouchable. The massaging of emollients should be beneficial and it may also reduce irritation produced by inflammatory and neural mechanisms.

Countering the hostile environment

The house dust mite's excrement plays a part in atopic eczema so one should try to reduce the population within the home. However, the expense and disruption has to be kept within acceptable limits. Methods include:

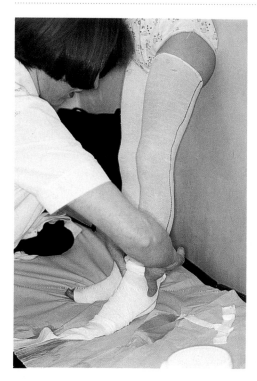

Fig. 78 Wet wraps.

- keeping the house well ventilated
- dusting using a wet cloth
- frequent vacuuming
- replace carpet with lino tiles
- consider dust-proof covers for mattresses and pillows.

Using cotton sheets and blankets permits better temperature regulation than a duvet [28]. Increasing the humidity in the home is

---

Indications for referral of atopic eczema to a specialist [29]
- diagnostic doubt
- failure to respond to maintenance treatment with mildly potent steroids in children or moderately potent steroids in adults
- second-line treatment required or dietary manipulation being tried
- when specialist opinion would be valuable in counselling patients and family

---

beneficial either by using a humidifier or simply bowls of water in the bedroom. Animal dander has an aggravating role and it is better to give advice early on to keep a goldfish, rather than later suggest the demise of an established Fido or Whiskers. If the family do keep a furry pet then it is best kept out of the child's bedroom.

Systemic therapies for severe atopic eczema
- Phototherapy.
- Photochemotherapy.
- Cyclosporin.
- Oral steroids.

Contact dermatitis

In a case of allergic contact dermatitis avoidance of allergens when possible is paramount. If this is impossible then exposure to the allergen should be minimized. With contact irritant eczema the patient should reduce the exposure to irritants and wear protective clothing. Examples of weak irritants are water, saline, weak acids, weak alkalis, soap, detergents, soluble oils and detergents. Stronger irritants are bleach, paraffin, white spirit, petroleum and caustics. The GP has to know the type, concentration and quantity of irritant the patient has been exposed to. Patients who have had atopic eczema are at risk of developing an irritant dermatitis. They should therefore avoid careers where their hands would frequently be in water or exposed to irritants.

Occupations at risk of irritant dermatitis
- bar staff
- catering and cleaning
- construction work
- engineering and mechanics
- farming and horticulture
- hairdressing
- nursing

In treating dermatitis exposure to irritants should be minimized and the use of protective gloves encouraged. Nappy rash is a common form of irritant dermatitis which responds to exposing the perineum to air. Asteototic eczema is another form of irritant eczema which responds to emollients.

Hand eczema

This is often a mixed bag as many patients may have a past history of atopy and a recent history of exposure to irritants. Any contact irritant or allergen should be excluded. If this is not possible then protective clothing should be worn, e.g. gloves.

Acute hand eczema, including pompholyx
It is worth prescribing potassium permanganate soaks and a course of oral antibiotic, e.g. flucloxacillin. After the soaks a potent topical steroid cream can be applied. Treatment of acute hand eczema includes:
• avoidance of irritants and allergens
• potassium permanganate soaks
• potent topical steroids with topical or oral antibiotics.

Chronic hand eczema
Chronic hand eczema requires the frequent use of emollients. Any irritant should be avoided wherever possible. Antibiotic steroid combinations can be helpful with cases of subacute eczema. Treatment of chronic hand eczema includes:
• avoidance of irritants and allergens
• emollients
• moderate potency steroid.

Other eczemas and related conditions

Infantile seborrhoeic eczema
The condition is self-limiting. For the scalp a tar shampoo, or a tar, salicylic acid and coconut shampoo can be used. For the napkin area, a hydrocortisone and imidazole combination product is effective, e.g. miconazole–hydrocortisone cream.

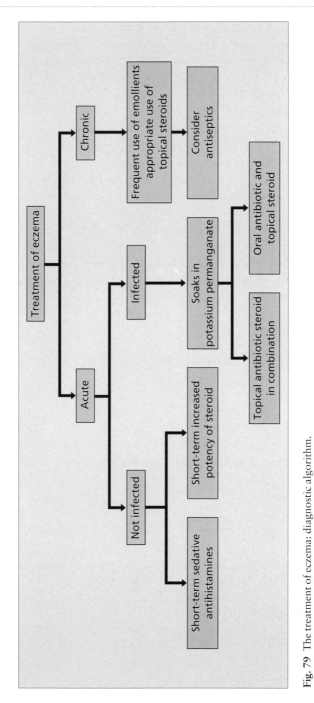

Fig. 79 The treatment of eczema: diagnostic algorithm.

Adult seborrhoeic eczema

The same preparations as for infantile seborrhoeic eczema can be used to treat adult seborrhoeic eczema. It is worth also considering ketoconazole cream and shampoo.

Discoid eczema

Discoid eczema usually needs a fairly potent steroid together with the treatment of any secondary infection. Treatments include:

* topical steroids of either moderate or strong potency
* topical antibiotics in combination with the steroid
* oral antibiotics with topical steroids
* emollients.

Varicose eczema

At this delicate site only a weak or moderate potency steroid should be prescribed. Topical antibiotics should be avoided because of the risk of sensitization. Appropriate support stockings are beneficial.

Lichen simplex

* Potent steroids.
* Emollients.

Pityriasis alba

* Reassurance.
* Emollients.

Juvenile plantar dermatosis

* Tar preparations.
* Emollients.
* Topical steroids.
* Reduce wearing of trainers.

The algorithm on p. 123 can be used as a guide to treating eczema (Fig. 79).

14 Management of psoriasis

There is no cure for psoriasis; however, it is possible to reduce both the extent and severity of the rash, if not clear it. When a patient presents with psoriasis the GP needs to know:

- how motivated they are as regarding treatment
- what effect the condition has on their quality of life
- the type, extent and severity of their psoriasis
- what home facilities and support they have.

A treatment plan should be developed for each individual patient. They may need a shampoo for their scalp, a vitamin D derivative for their plaques on elbows and knees and a weak steroid antimicrobial for the flexures.

Points to discuss at initial presentation are as follows [30]
- explanation of psoriasis, including reassurance that it is neither infectious nor malignant
- treatment options (including no active treatment)
- the probable benefit the patient can expect from treatment
- techniques of application of any topical treatment (especially important with dithranol and scalp preparations)
- introduction to patient support groups, e.g. Psoriasis Association and the Psoriatic Arthropathy Alliance

Types of psoriasis

Scalp psoriasis

Those with mild scalp involvement find a shampoo acceptable. When there is more severe involvement other therapies are necessary. A potent steroid lotion used each morning is a cosmetically acceptable treatment. An alternative is a vitamin D scalp solution used twice daily. For those with severe involvement an ointment containing tar, salicylic acid and coconut oil is effective. This is left on for 1 hour and then washed off. It may be necessary to use a combination of these therapies to treat a range of patients and scalps.

Plaque psoriasis of the trunk and limbs
A vitamin D derivative is a cosmetically acceptable first-line therapy. If irritation is a problem this can be overcome by alternating a moderate potency steroid with the vitamin D analogue. Calcipotriol in combination with a topical steroid may clear psoriasis for patients who are low responders to calcipotriol alone [31]. For patients who do not respond one can consider dithranol or a topical retinoid. Because of the risk of local side effects potent steroids should not be first-line therapy. Tachyphylaxis can develop to topical steroids and they can make psoriasis unstable.

Topical therapy for psoriasis		
Therapy	Advantages	Disadvantages
Emollients	Simple	Limited effect
Vitamin D derivatives	Effective	Irritation
Tar	Simple	Acceptability and odour
Topical steroids	Acceptability	Potential local and systemic side effects
Vitamin A derivatives	Acceptability	Irritation
Dithranol	Effective	Time, mess and irritation

Localized pustular psoriasis of the hands and feet
One might try a potent steroid, a vitamin D derivative or topical tar. However, these cases are difficult to treat and referral to secondary care is often necessary.

Guttate psoriasis
Sometimes an emollient is all that is required. Tar is an effective therapy, or a moderate potency steroid alternated with topical calcipotriol. If the rash does not clear referral to secondary care for UVB should be considered.

Flexural psoriasis
Many treatments used on plaque psoriasis on the trunk and limbs irritate when used in the flexures. Caused by the warm moist environment of the flexures, secondary infection is common. The flexures are also a site very prone to steroid-induced side effects. A weak or moderate potency steroid is therefore often used in com-

bination with an antimicrobial. Vitamin D derivatives can be tried in the flexures but there may be irritation.

Facial psoriasis

An emollient is worth trying and if this is not effective then treat as flexural psoriasis. Psoriasis of the face and flexures is difficult to treat and there is little alternative to topical steroids. These are the very sites susceptible to steroid atrophy and so only a weak or moderate potency steroid is used. Tar and vitamin D derivatives can be tried although irritation often limits their use.

Nail deformity caused by psoriasis

Patients should keep the nails short and try to avoid trauma to the nails. There is no effective topical treatment, although various steroids and topical vitamin D derivatives have been tried. Systemic therapies can improve the nail dystrophy; however, they are rarely indicated for this alone.

Psoriasis and quality of life

The effect of a chronic skin disease on the patient's quality of life should not be forgotten and the need to treat more than the epidermis should be remembered. Psoriasis is correlated with high levels of anxiety and depression, and a concomitant oral antidepressant can improve the results of topical therapies [32].

Indications for referral to a consultant dermatologist [33]
- diagnostic difficulty
- request for patient counselling or education, or both, including initial demonstration of topical treatment
- failure of topical treatment used appropriately for 3 months
- need for increasing amounts or potencies of topical corticosteroids
- need for systemic drugs
- generalized pustular or erythrodermic psoriasis (emergency referral)

One of the earliest forms of treatment involving a systemic therapy was described by Ingram in 1953. This consisted of tar baths, ultraviolet radiation and 24 h treatment with increasing concentrations of dithranol in Lassar's paste [34].

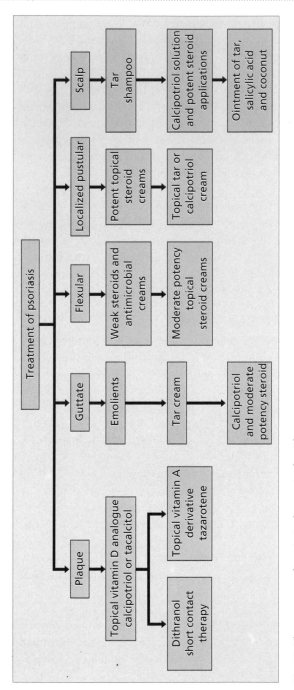

Fig. 80 The treatment of psoriasis: diagnostic algorithm.

Systemic therapies for severe psoriasis
- Phototherapy—either broad- or narrow-band UVB.
- Photochemotherapy—PUVA using UVA with oral or bath psoralens.
- Methotrexate.
- Oral retinoids.
- Cyclosporin.

Lichen planus
- Patient usually under secondary care.
- Potent and very potent steroids.
- Oral steroids.

Pityriasis rosea
- Advice only.
- Calamine lotion.
- Weak potency steroids.
- Aqueous cream with 1% menthol.

When deciding on treatment of psoriasis the algorithm on p. 128 can be used (Fig. 80).

15 Management of flexural, hair and nail problems

The flexures

When treating flexural rashes the skin is moist and oozing, therefore creams rather than ointments are used. As there is no thick scale with conditions in this area there is no need to use potent topical steroids. Indeed potent steroids should be avoided in the flexures because of the increased risk of side effects in this rather closed moist environment.

Secondary infection is common in the flexures. Patients may require combination products, as dual pathology is often present. If fungal infections are being treated, then it is important that the patient completes the therapy or relapse will follow. A topical imidazole is suitable for treating dermatophyte or candidal infections. This, in combination with 1% hydrocortisone, is also suitable for treating psoriasis and eczema at this site. Resistant or extensive fungal disease may require systemic therapy.

Anal irritation

Anal hygiene needs to be improved, and the use of soft toilet paper should be encouraged. If possible the anal area should be washed after defaecation, avoiding soap as this produces irritation. A bidet is ideal, but a large bowl or a bath are alternatives. One should discourage aggressive wiping which produces trauma. The skin should be dried carefully by dabbing gently with a towel or soft tissue. Loose fitting underpants help to reduce the humidity or, perhaps even better, changing to highland dress is to be recommended!

Hidradenitis suppurativa
- Similar to the treatment of acne.
- Oral antibiotics.
- Topical antiseptics.
- Surgery—excision.

Hyperhydrosis
- Topical 20% aluminium chloride.
- Iontophoresis.
- Oral anticholinergics.
- Surgery.

Lichen sclerosus et atrophicus
- Usually under secondary care.
- Potent topical steroids.
- Aqueous cream.

The scalp

The scalp is not an easy site to treat, as it can be quite hairy! Shampoos are easy to use, but have the therapeutic pitfall of a short contact time with the involved skin. Applications and lotions are clean and acceptable, but those in alcoholic bases tend to sting if the scalp is excoriated. Patients find ointments greasy and messy but they are effective.

Patients can combine different therapies, applying Cocois ointment in the early evening, which they then wash out, and a steroid or vitamin D analogue lotion which they apply each morning. There is less risk of local side effects from topical steroids applied to the scalp than there is on the face and flexures. Topical steroids are available in various formulations, some in combination with salicylic acid. Not all scalp therapies are only available on the NHS, some are only available on private prescription.

Scalp conditions covered in other sections
- Seborrhoeic eczema (p. 122).
- Psoriasis (p. 125).
- Tinea capitis (p. 136–138).

Alopecia areata
- Advice only.
- Intralesional triamcinolone.
- Wigs.
- Irritants and induced contact allergic dermatitis.

Androgenetic alopecia
- Advice only.
- Topical minoxidil liquid (not on NHS).
- Oral Finasteride (only for male patients and in certain countries, e.g. the USA).

Hirsutism
- Shaving.
- Waxing.
- Bleaching.
- Ethinyloestradiol/cyproterone acetate.

The nails

- Fungal infections—covered in other sections (see pp. 137–138).
- Psoriasis—no treatment, rarely systemic therapies, screen for secondary fungal infection.
- Trauma—chiropody.
- Lichen planus—no treatment, rarely systemic therapies.
- Alopecia areata—no treatment.

16 Urticaria and rashes without surface scale

Urticaria

Acute urticaria is not uncommon and frequently just needs symptomatic treatment with oral antihistamines. Sometimes there is a history of eating strawberries or taking penicillin and these should then be avoided in the future.

Short-lived episodes of urticaria can be controlled by taking a short-acting non-sedative antihistamine as required. If the disease is chronic it is worth the patient taking a non-sedative antihistamine on a regular basis. Drugs, such as aspirin, can cause an exacerbation in up to 40% of patients and they should be advised not to take them. After being symptom-free from urticaria the patient then omits the antihistamine to see if they relapse. If one non-sedating antihistamine does not control symptoms after a couple of weeks it is worth switching to another. Some patients taking a non-sedative antihistamine benefit from the addition of a sedative antihistamine at night. Topical steroids have no effect on urticaria.

> Non-sedative antihistamines for adults with urticaria
> - cetirizine 10 mg daily
> - loratadine 10 mg daily
> - fexofenadine 180 mg daily

Parenteral adrenaline, hydrocortisone and antihistamines may be required in cases of anaphylaxis and angioedema which involve the mouth and tongue. Cases of hereditary C1 esterase inhibitor deficiency may require fresh frozen plasma.

Rashes without surface scale

Granuloma annulare
- Advice only.
- Potent topical steroids to active edge.

Morphoea
- Advice only.
- Topical steroids.

Vitiligo
- Advice on sun exposure.
- Sunscreens.
- Cosmetic camouflage.

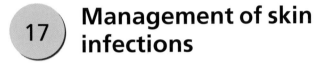

Management of skin infections

17

Bacterial infections

Impetigo is usually caused by *Staphylococcus aureus* and occasionally by *Streptococcus pyogenes*. Impetigo is highly infectious and patients should use their own towel and soap. Small areas of impetigo can be treated with topical antibiotics, such as either fusidic acid or mupirocin. More extensive areas or multiple lesions require a systemic antibiotic, e.g. flucloxacillin or erythromycin. An acute paronychia is usually caused by *S. aureus*. The patient can be advised to soak his or her finger in warm saline for 15 min, then gently probe the nail-fold; frequently and painlessly pus bursts through. A course of oral antibiotic can then be prescribed.

Erysipelas/cellulitis
Streptococcus pyogenes is the usual pathogen and the treatment is a systemic antibiotic, usually high-dose penicillin. Those who are ill require hospital admission and parenteral penicillin. Certainly in primary care it is worth considering giving the first dose of penicillin by intramuscular injection at the time of consultation. Patients with recurrent cellulitis of a limb need prolonged courses of antibiotics. Any coexistent tinea pedis which acted as a portal of entry for bacteria needs treatment.

Erythrasma
- Oral erythromycin.
- Topical fusidic acid.
- Topical miconazole.

Pitted keratolysis
- Potassium permanganate soaks.
- Oral erythromycin.
- Topical fusidic acid.
- Foot hygiene.

Superficial fungal infections

Many minor fungal infections respond to a simple topical antifungal therapy, such as an imidazole cream, which can be purchased at the local pharmacy.

Yeast infections

Candida is a unicellular yeast which is implicated in nappy rash and intertrigo. An imidazole cream provides a suitable treatment. With a nappy rash the area should be exposed to the air and for intertrigo the flexural surfaces need to be separated. Candida is one of the major factors in a chronic paronychia. Clotrimazole lotion should be applied along the nail-fold and the patient instructed to keep the hands as dry as possible.

The Pityrosporum yeast causes pityriasis versicolor. An imidazole cream can be used to treat small areas; patients with an extensive rash can be treated with 200 mg of oral itraconazole for 1 week. The Pityrosporum yeast is implicated in seborrhoeic dermatitis and keto-conazole cream and shampoo are effective therapies.

Treatment of dermatophyte infections

Many minor dermatophyte infections, such as athlete's foot, respond to a topical imidazole cream. Topical terbinafine may be tried in difficult cases as it is more effective than topical imidazoles, although it is more expensive. When treating tinea pedis all the toe web spaces should be inspected and all those involved treated. Resistant cases can be treated with oral terbinafine or itraconazole. Athlete's foot tends to be spread by communal bathing and showers. If there is difficulty in clearing superficial fungal infections one should be suspicious of nail involvement acting as a reservoir of infection. Tinea cruris is another common fungal skin infection. When treating tinea cruris it should be remembered that coexistent tinea pedis is highly likely and also needs treatment.

> Systemic antifungal therapy is required when
> - the rash is extensive
> - the rash is resistant to topical therapy
> - the scalp is involved
> - treating fungal nail disease

Tinea capitis needs an oral therapy, such as griseofulvin, and concomitant use of a topical antifungal, e.g. ketoconazole shampoo, will reduce the spread of infection. A minor infection of one or two nails can be treated with weekly amorolfine nail lacquer. However, most cases are too extensive or severe for a topical therapy and require a systemic agent. When treating fungal nail disease successful patient management will depend on making a correct diagnosis, and taking into account the risk/benefit ratio of any treatment that is considered [35].

Those interested in treating fungal nail disease should read the report from the British Society for Medical Mycology [36].

The summary points of the report were:
- onychomycosis is usually caused by dermatophytes (85–90%), but several fungi that are difficult to treat affect toe-nails
- paronychia is caused by many *Candida* species, some resistant to azole drugs
- samples for mycology should be taken as proximally as possible in the nail
- demonstration of hyphae in a nail specimen by microscopy is sufficient to start treatment
- choice of treatment depends on many factors, including patient's age and preference, infecting fungus, number of nails affected, degree of nail involvement, whether toe-nails or finger-nails are infected, and other drugs being taken

Griseofulvin has low cure rates when treating fungal nail infections, unlike terbinafine which is a highly effective therapy for dermatophyte nail infections. Pulsed itraconazole is an alternative and has the advantage that it can be used to treat both dermatophyte and yeast nail infections. Patients should be advised that the fungicidal therapy kills the fungus, then after cessation of therapy the diseased nail containing fungus continues to grow out over many months.

Treatment of fungal nail disease			
	Griseofulvin	Terbinafine	Itraconazole
Dosage	500 mg daily	250 mg daily	200 mg b.d. one week a month
Finger-nails	6 months	6 weeks	One pulse of therapy
Toe-nails	18 months	12 weeks	Three pulses of therapy

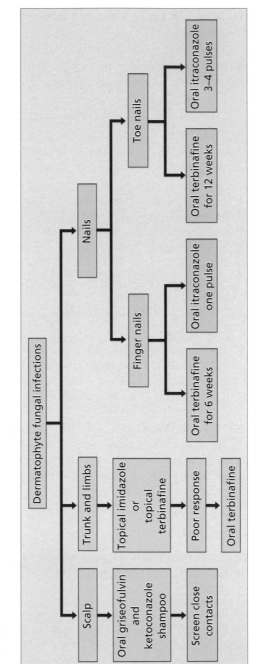

Fig. 81 The treatment of tinea: diagnostic algorithm.

The algorithm on p. 138 guides the reader through treatment choices for tinea (Fig. 81).

Viral infections

There are a whole host of viral infections which can infect the skin. Many viral infections are self limiting and do not need active treatment. The risks, inconvenience and expense of any treatment must be balanced against its benefits.

Warts

Viral warts are a common self-limiting problem in primary care and the more patients one treats, the more will present. If viral warts remain untreated approximately one-third will resolve within 6 months and two-thirds in 2 years [37]. On hearing this explanation patients and their families frequently decide on no treatment and await spontaneous resolution. Treatment, if any, depends on the site and type of wart. For those who do require treatment there are a variety of paints, gels and cryotherapy.

When treating viral warts remember [11]
- up to 80% respond to paints and gels in 100 treatment days
- plane warts on the face are best left untreated
- warts unresponsive to conservative treatment may be treated with cryosurgery
- cryosurgery is very painful and not well tolerated by children
- mosaic plantar warts are often resistant to cryosurgery
- curettage of warts may result in scarring

Common warts and verrucae

Warts and verrucae abound and if left alone will disappear without scarring. There is little point trying to treat a patient with multiple warts; the warts will frequently spread faster than they can be treated. However, some believe treating a few warts can induce an immune response which affects all the other warts.

Keratolytics, such as salicylic acid and lactic acid, have a place. It is important to pare warts down before treating. Patients who do use treatment must follow the advice leaflets which come with the various preparations. The usual problem is irritation, which resolves if treatment is withheld for a few days.

Other warts

Facial warts should be left alone or treated with cryotherapy. Plane warts rarely respond to any therapy. A topical retinoid can be tried but does not have a product licence for this indication. Mosaic warts are very difficult to treat; soaks using gluteraldehyde can be tried. The normal tissue is protected with Vaseline while the mosaic wart is soaked in a 10% solution of gluteraldehyde. This involves both time and motivation. Patients should be advised that there can be staining of the skin. Podophyllum is no more effective than salicylic acid, should not be used in pregnancy and is probably best left in the hands of secondary care.

Cryosurgery has its place but it does have the potential to inflict pain, suffering and scarring. Children who do not want or need treatment should not undergo pain and suffering at their parents' behest. Genital warts are a special case, and these patients are best referred to a urogenital clinic where screening for other diseases can be performed.

Molluscum contagiosum

These benign lesions will resolve spontaneously and no active treatment is advised. If there is a desire to treat actively, then anything which disrupts the papules speeds clearance. Gentle cryotherapy in experienced hands is quite effective.

Herpes simplex

Herpes simplex can cause some discomfort and anxiety. The use of sunscreens can reduce repeated attacks. Many cases do not require any active treatment; however, therapies available include topical and oral aciclovir and topical penciclovir.

Topical antivirals for herpes simplex		
Indication	Aciclovir cream	Penciclovir cream
Herpes simplex	4 hourly	2 hourly

There are a range of antivirals creating various treatment options. For treatment of an acute attack to be effective it has to be started

early. Long-term prescribing of antivirals can prevent recurrence; however, there are cost implications.

Oral antivirals for herpes simplex			
Indication	Aciclovir	Valaciclovir	Famciclovir
Herpes labialis	200 mg 5 times day		
Genital initial	200 mg 5 times day	500 mg b.d.	250 mg t.d.s.
Herpes recurrent	200 mg 5 times day	500 mg b.d.	125 mg b.d.
Prevention	400 mg b.d.		250 mg b.d.

Herpes zoster (shingles)

Patients with active shingles are shedding the virus. For treatment to modify the disease process it has to be given early. Any zoster affecting the head and neck, especially the eye, needs prompt intervention with provision of the appropriate therapy.

Systemic treatment of shingles in adults		
Aciclovir	Valaciclovir	Famciclovir
800 mg 5 times a day	500 mg b.d. for 5–10 days	750 mg daily for 7 days

The elderly are a group especially at risk of developing post-herpetic neuralgia and should be considered for early active treatment. Treatments available include oral aciclovir, valaciclovir and famciclovir.

Patients with immunodeficiency

Patients with any immunodeficiency need early intensive treatment of infections. The dosage of drug can be higher and one should consult more detailed literature.

Infestations

Head lice

Head lice infestation is on the increase, as are the requests for medication. If the GP is going to prescribe medication then the local policy should be followed. In the best interests of all concerned, the frequent use of nit combs should become the mainstay of treatment. It is possible to suffocate the nits with Vaseline; however, washing it out is a very difficult task.

> In the treatment of head lice
> - only those with active infestation need treatment
> - one can clear infection by physical means
> - there is anxiety over safety of insecticides
> - there is an increasing number of resistant strains to insecticides

Scabies

It is vital to treat *all* close contacts and this may need some detective work. All those receiving treatment must follow the instruction leaflets enclosed with their treatment. Work involving conscientious objectors in the Second World War proved that you need close body contact to spread scabies.

A suitable scabicide is a 5% permethrin cream which is applied over the whole body and washed off after 8 hours. The bed linen and clothing need laundering and patients should be advised that the itch continues for up to 4 weeks after treatment. Failure of treatment is a result of either inappropriate use of treatment or failure to treat all those involved. If a single treatment does not succeed, then everyone should be treated twice with permethrin cream, with a 4-day gap between applications. Special attention should be paid to treating the flexures, genitalia and under the nails. If the hands are washed before the first 8 hours after application of cream, repeat the application of scabicide to this site.

18 Management of leg ulcers

Treatment of chronic venous ulceration includes:
- wound cleaning and dressing
- compression bandages
- leg elevation
- exercises.

The leg ulcer needs cleaning and dressing, with the initial removal of any clot, debris and necrotic tissue. The ulcer can be washed with saline and, if infected, soaked in potassium permanganate solution. Long-term antiseptics, however, may reduce wound healing so are not used routinely. The dressing depends upon the state of the ulcer. For those cases with a heavy exudate an alginate, which is highly absorbent, is appropriate. If there is a light or moderate exudate then a hydrocolloid is suitable. No topical antibiotics are used on leg ulcers as these can produce contact allergic reactions.

If the ulcer is dry, then a non-adherent dressing can be used. The frequency of changing dressings depends upon the amount of exudate the ulcer is producing at that particular time. Any associated varicose eczema should be treated with weak or moderate potency topical steroid. More potent steroids should be avoided if possible because of their potential local side effects.

Once arterial disease has been excluded the venous hypertension needs to be treated by graduated compressive bandaging; crepe bandages are not sufficient. Patients need to use support stockings long-term after healing. Leg elevation should be encouraged and leg exercises taught. Any coexistent problem such as anaemia, cardiac failure or oedema from any cause needs treatment. A social history is required, with a home visit from a member of the team to assess accommodation and support.

Ulcers are colonized by many bacteria which need no treatment. However, if the wound is malodorous with erythema, it may have become infected. The spreading infection can produce erysipelas and a bacteraemia. The patient develops a fever and experiences pain.

If the ulcer is infected then it is worth taking a swab and prescribing
- penicillin for *Streptococcus pyogenes* infection
- flucloxacillin for *Staphylococcus aureus* infection
- metronidazole for *Bacteroides* infection

Progress of patients with leg ulcers should be monitored. Each patient with a leg ulcer should have one key member of staff to follow them up. Objective assessment can be obtained by tracing the ulcer in difficult cases. Those patients most at risk of poor healing are those who:
- have had an ulcer for more than 5 years
- have other major medical problems
- are immobile or live alone.

If there is delayed healing of a leg ulcer one should consider:
- whether initial diagnosis correct
- change in general medical state
- poor compliance to treatment
- social and domestic circumstances of patient
- any evidence of malignant change in ulcer.

Formulations

Topical or systemic therapy

Topical therapies avoid the risks, side effects and possible drug inter-actions of systemic therapies. They are therefore often preferred in primary care. The site of a rash affects its suitability for topical therapy. Diseases which are deeper in the skin, e.g. in the subcuta-neous tissues, require a systemic therapy. An extensive rash can be difficult to treat with a topical therapy. If one wishes to suppress a rash whose site is unpredictable, e.g. urticaria, then a topical therapy would be inappropriate.

Overcoming the skin's barrier
The skin acts as a barrier to the absorption of topical therapies. This barrier is reduced in inflammatory skin disorders and more drug is absorbed through the damaged skin compared to normal skin. The flexures are a site of increased hydration which results in increased absorption of topical therapies. The palms and soles have a thick stratum corneum reducing the absorption of topical therapies.

How the drug gets through
Some topical therapies are better absorbed than others. Drugs of low molecular size are more easily absorbed. Those which are hydro-philic are more easily absorbed through the stratum corneum, and those which are lipophilic pass more easily through cell membranes.

One can increase the absorption of a drug by
- increasing its concentration up to a maximum
- hydrating the stratum corneum
- using occlusion
- increasing the temperature

Duration of therapy
With an active inflammatory dermatosis the skin's barrier function is reduced and more topical therapy is absorbed. Topical therapies tend

to pool in the epidermis which acts as a reservoir from where they are released. This means that the duration of action is much longer than the duration of application.

A bactericidal or fungicidal therapy can be given for a shorter length of time than a bacteriostatic or fungistatic therapy. Infections in the subcutaneous tissues, such as a cellulitis, can require a prolonged course of systemic antibiotic therapy. Fungal nail infections need longer courses of therapy than fungal skin infections.

Health economics

Health economics is a major issue these days. Sometimes the GP has to consider more than the unit cost of a drug, which has little relationship to its cost-effectiveness [38]. One has to consider not only the quantity of topical preparations used, but also their frequency of application and the duration of treatment required to produce a desired effect. Not only is there the cost of treating a patient in primary care, but also the cost of secondary referral and treatment.

Volumes

The GP needs to advise how much of a preparation should be applied and make sure that sufficient treatment has been used as prescribed. Labels on cartons stating apply twice daily leave much to the patient's imagination. To perform one application of cream or ointment to an adult's body requires 30 g. Invariably treatments such as

A guide to quantity (g) of cream or ointment required for twice daily applications for one week [39]			
Age	Whole body	Arms and legs	Trunk
6 months	35	20	15
1 year	45	25	15
4 years	60	35	20
8 years	90	50	35
12 years	120	65	45
16 years	155	85	55
Adult (70 kg male)	170	90	60

Adapted with permission from Hunter, J.A.A., Savin, J.A. & Dahl, M.V. (1995) *Clinical Dermatology* (2nd edn), p. 281, Blackwell Science, Oxford.

emollients are underprescribed. They need to be supplied in adequate quantities, e.g. volumes of 500 g.

Fingertip units

If a cream or ointment is squeezed out of a tube with a standard 5 mm nozzle over the distal section of an adult's index finger the amount equates to approximately 0.5 g. This is a fingertip unit (FTU) and 2 FTU should cover the area of the flat of four hands [40].

The fingertip unit	
Site for an adult	Quantity (FTU)
Face and neck	2.5
Front and back of trunk	14
One arm	3
One hand, both sides	1
One leg	6
One foot	2

One must remember that fingertip units relate to an adult's finger and palm. Fingertip units are a safe guide to the amount of topical steroid required to treat eczema [41].

Formulations

It is necessary for the topical medication to be in a formulation which makes it suitable to treat the rash in question and is acceptable to the patient. The most appropriate vehicle or base depends on the site and type of rash. For acute rashes a lotion or cream is preferable, while for chronic dry scaly rash an ointment is best. Patients do not like greasy preparations on the face and prefer creams. The flexures are moist and a cream is the preferred vehicle. Patients in a warm climate also prefer to use cream formulations.

Soaks

Potassium permanganate soaks are useful for treating acute infections. The crystals can be dissolved in a small quantity in water to produce a light pink solution.

Shampoo
Shampoos are useful for treating scalp problems. As they only have a short contact time they are only suitable for mild scalp problems.

Lotion
Lotions are a liquid formulation, either in water or alcohol. They have to be applied frequently and have a cooling effect, which can be useful on acutely inflamed oozing eruptions. Shake lotions have powder added which tends to make them clump and are not very acceptable.

Paint
Paints can be used to apply a topical treatment to nails.

Gel
Gels are transparent semi-solid emulsions which tend to become a liquid on contact with a warm surface. They are suitable for treating scalp problems.

Cream
Creams hydrate the skin and increase absorption of other compounds. However, the evaporation of water after application of a cream tends to have a paradoxical drying effect. Creams spread more easily than ointments and tend to be more cosmetically acceptable. They are suitable for the face, flexures and palms, and are used in acute and subacute conditions. Because creams have a high water content they need preservatives which can cause sensitization.

Ointment
Ointments are greasier than creams, and when applied to the skin form an occlusive layer. They tend to be more effective than creams and last longer. Ointments are useful in chronic conditions. One thinks of ointments as inert bases; however, white soft paraffin has anti-inflammatory properties. The pharmaceutical industry tries to make preparations which have the beneficial properties of an ointment, combined with the cosmetic acceptability of a cream. This can be done; however, someone has to foot the bill!

Powder

Powders can be used in moist areas, such as the flexures, although creams are probably more acceptable.

Paste

A paste is an ointment base with added powder to produce a stiff preparation. A paste gets the active drug to the required site and reduces the spread to surrounding area.

20 Specific therapies in detail

Emollients

Emollients provide a very safe therapy for many conditions, such as dry skin, eczema and psoriasis. They form a film over the skin, smoothing out the contours and reducing loss of fluid. They hydrate the skin and help restore its normal barrier function. If emollients are applied before other topical therapies they can make them more effective.

An emollient can be prescribed as a cream, ointment, bath emollient and soap substitute. Patient preference is important, and they must be willing to use the emollient prescribed. The more expensive the emollient the more cosmetically acceptable it is, rather than it being more efficacious. While the best emollient is the one the patient will use, the physician has to accept that funds are limited and prescribing must be evidence based.

Patients can use different emollients at different sites; a cream may be used on the face and palms where a less greasy preparation is preferred, and an ointment which is more effective would be used for other sites. Different emollients can be used at different times of the day. A cosmetically acceptable cream may be used in the morning and a thicker ointment at night. The major problem with emollients is that they are not used sufficiently often. Patients can have a small pot of emollient to carry around with them to use frequently. Patients will only use an emollient that they find cosmetically acceptable and then this needs to be prescribed in adequate quantities.

Examples of emollients

Aqueous cream is a 'thin' emollient, oily cream can be regarded as a standard emollient, and white soft paraffin is a thicker emollient. Although oily cream is inexpensive it does contain lanolin which can occasionally cause sensitization.

Aqueous cream or emulsifying ointment can be prescribed as soap substitutes. Emulsifying ointment is an inexpensive emollient; however, it does make the bath slippery, so do advise care and the use of a bath mat. Patients can mix their own bath emollient by mixing two tablespoons of emulsifying ointment in a blender with a pint of water; this makes a creamy mixture which can be used in the bath [42].

Topical steroids

Topical steroids reduce inflammation and are used to treat the common inflammatory dermatoses, such as eczema and psoriasis. They are also used in discoid lupus erythematosus and lichen planus.

Potency of topical steroids
Topical steroids are available in a range of potencies including weak, moderate, potent and very potent preparations. Hydrocortisone is the weakest steroid, and modification to the steroid molecule, such as fluorination, increases its potency. Urea in combination with a topical steroid converts a weak into a moderate potency.

Potency of topical steroids			
Mild	Moderate	Potent	Very potent
Hydrocortisone 1%	Clobetasone butyrate 0.05%	Betamethasone 0.1% valerate	Clobetasol proprionate 0.05%
Hydrocortisone 2.5%	Fluocortolone hexanoate 0.25%	Mometasone furoate 0.1%	Halcinonide 0.1%

One can either start with:
- a weak steroid and increase the potency if there is no improvement
- start with a more potent steroid and then reduce the potency.

If one starts with a more potent steroid then one gains quicker control and probably uses less steroid in the long term. However, there is a danger that the patient will not reduce the potency as required. Inflamed skin does absorb steroid more easily, and this absorption does reduce as the rash improves. Therefore inflamed skin should be quite responsive to low potency steroids. Tachyphylaxis can develop to topical steroids in long-term use and changing the steroid molecule is beneficial.

Parents are often worried about thinning of their children's skin as a result of application of topical steroids. It is reasonable to prescribe 1% hydrocortisone ointment as required to control infantile eczema. Educating and informing patients on steroid potencies is well worthwhile. The risk of side effects from mild potency steroids are low. It would be unusual for more than a moderate potency steroid to be used for atopic eczema in practice. Very potent steroids are reserved for problems such as:

- inflammatory dermatoses on palms and soles
- lichen planus
- discoid lupus erythematosus.

The site of application of topical steroid

Different sites and different age groups can tolerate different potencies. The stratum corneum is thicker on the palms and soles and can tolerate potent steroids, while the thinner skin on the face should be treated with weak steroids. In the flexures there is increased hydration and scale is reduced; weak steroids should be used at this site. The stratum corneum is thinner on children and in the elderly.

Side effects of topical steroids

Side effects from topical steroids are either local at the site of action or systemic. Local side effects include thinning of the skin, bruising and striae (Fig. 82). Rashes can develop, including acne, rosacea and perioral dermatitis. Areas of hypopigmentation can develop at the site of application of topical steroids. There can be an exacerbation of superficial skin infections and the nature of a rash can be modified, making diagnosis more difficult, e.g. tinea incognito. Systemic side effects include Cushing's syndrome, suppression of the pituitary–adrenal axis. The side effects from topical steroids are related to:

- the age of the patient
- site of treatment
- potency of steroid used
- the duration of treatment
- the quantity used
- if occlusion is used
- if other medication is used in combination with the topical steroid.

While topical steroids have a major role in the treatment of eczema, in psoriasis their use should be limited to the face and flexures.

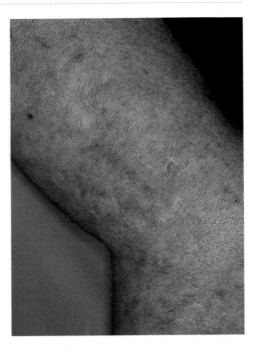

Fig. 82 Striae from topical steroids.

Safe average weekly dosage of topical steroids for adults [43]			
Duration of treatment (months)	Mild–moderate (g)	Potent (g)	Very potent (g)
< 2	100	50	30
2–6	50	30	15
6–12	25	15	7.5

Reproduced from [43] with permission.

Potent topical steroids can make plaque psoriasis unstable and are not used as first-line therapy in this condition.

Corticosteroids and immunosuppressants

Oral steroids
- Indications—bullous diseases and vasculitis.
- Rarely used in psoriasis and eczema.
- Erosive lichen planus.

Cyclosporin
- Indications include severe eczema and severe psoriasis.
- Monitor blood pressure and renal function.

Urea

Urea has an emollient effect and hydrates the stratum corneum. It enhances penetration of other agents.

Salicylic acid

Salicylic acid causes destruction of keratin and hence reduces scale. It can cause irritation and, very occasionally, hypersensitivity. Salicylic acid is used alone or in combination to treat psoriasis and seborrhoeic dermatitis. It can increase absorption of other drugs. There is anxiety about possible salicylate absorption in infants using salicylic acid on large areas. Increased concentrations of salicylic acid can be used to treat warts and callosities.

Antihistamines

Oral antihistamines fall into two broad groups, depending on whether they produce significant sedation. The reduced sedation of some antihistamines is because they do not cross the blood–brain barrier in significant amounts. Because of this they cannot have a major central action in reducing itch. The non-sedative antihistamines are therefore useful in treating urticaria and other allergic reactions, such as insect bites.

Non-sedative antihistamines
Examples of non-sedative antihistamines are acrivastine, cetirizine, loratadine and terfenadine. Some non-sedative antihistamines can produce cardiac problems, with QT prolongation leading to dangerous dysrhythmias. These risks occur in patients with either hepatic impairment or those taking other medications which are liver enzyme inhibitors, including the azole antifungals and macrolide

antibiotics. Terfenadine can cause problems, but these difficulties are overcome by using its active metabolite, fexofenadine.

Sedative antihistamines

Sedative antihistamines not only treat urticaria but reduce itch. They can therefore be prescribed to reduce the nocturnal itch associated with eczema. The benefit tends to be lost if these drugs are used long-term. Chlorpheniramine can be given orally for urticaria and it also reduces the pruritus associated with eczema. Chlorpheniramine is administered by injection in cases of anaphylaxis.

Vitamin D derivatives

Vitamin D has a beneficial effect on psoriasis. It reduces the increased cell turnover and improves the lack of cell differentiation. It is desirable to maximize the beneficial effects of topical vitamin D on the skin and minimize the effects on general calcium metabolism. Therefore topical vitamin D analogues have been developed.

Calcipotriol

Calcipotriol is the most widely investigated topical vitamin D derivative. It is a clean effective remedy for treating mild to moderate psoriasis long-term in primary care [44]. It can be used in cases with up to 40% of the body surface involved. The calcipotriol cream or ointment is applied twice daily to plaque psoriasis on the trunk and limbs. Improvement is visible at 2 weeks and continues for at least 8 weeks. It can cause transient irritation and rarely causes photosensitivity. There is a lotion formulation which can be used to treat scalp psoriasis.

The maximum quantity of calcipotriol is:
- children over 6 years 50 g weekly
- children over 12 years 75 g weekly
- a maximum of 100 g weekly for adults.

Tacalcitol

Tacalcitol is a vitamin D analogue which is used once daily and, unlike calcipotriol, can be applied to the face. One should not use more than 5 g daily, and the maximum duration of treatment is of two 12-week courses in a year. Calcipotriol used twice daily is more effective than tacalcitol once daily [45].

Vitamin A derivatives

Topical retinoids are used to treat acne. There is tretinoin, its isomer, isotretinoin, and the retinoid-like drug, adapalene. These are highly effective at treating comedones and adapalene also reduces inflammation. Tretinoin causes an initial flare of acne. Topical retinoids should be avoided in pregnancy because their oral counterparts are highly teratogenic.

Topical retinoids have also been found to have a beneficial effect on psoriasis, reducing the hyperproliferation and inflammation, and helping normalize the lack of cell differentiation. The topical retinoid tazarotene can be used to treat mild to moderate psoriasis on the trunk and limbs of adults with up to 10% of their body surface affected [46]. This drug is available in a gel formulation which is cosmetically acceptable. However, it can cause irritation and it should not be applied to the face. The gel is applied in the evening and the patient instructed to wash their hands afterwards. There is low systemic absorption and the drug's half-life is only 18 h. As a precaution, females are asked to use contraceptive measures. Therapy can be continued for up to 12 weeks.

Dithranol

Dithranol (anthralin) is a synthetic derivative of chrysarobin, which comes from the araroba tree. Dithranol is a very effective therapy for psoriasis. The traditional method was to add dithranol to Lassar's paste; however, this was quite messy and time consuming to apply. Newer formulations are available and more suited to primary care. Dithranol can cause irritation of the skin which can be severe; this tends to be worse for those with fair skin and hair. It is not really suitable for the face, scalp and flexures. Dithranol can cause brown staining of the skin.

Short contact therapy with dithranol can be performed in the patient's home. The inflamed skin presents less of a barrier than normal skin and a reservoir of the drug can accumulate in the stratum corneum. A proprietary cream, ointment or wax stick is used, as these are more cosmetically acceptable. The dithranol is carefully applied to plaques on trunk and limbs. It is left for approximately 30 min and then washed off using a liquid soap. Increasing strengths of dithranol are used, starting with 0.1% and increasing to 2%. The patient needs to wash his or her hands thoroughly after each application and also clean the bath or shower tray afterwards. Practical demonstrations and patient advice leaflets are helpful.

Tar

Tar is a very old remedy which has anti-inflammatory properties. Coal can be distilled to produce coal tar which can be further refined to obtain purified preparations. Crude extracts of tar are available in white or yellow soft paraffin. The more purified tar preparations are available as creams, which are more cosmetically acceptable with little loss of efficacy.

Tar can be used to treat psoriasis, atopic eczema and scalp seborrhoeic dermatitis. Juvenile plantar dermatosis is a condition which responds to topical tar. Tar can cause irritation, an acneform rash and occasionally a folliculitis. Tar can rarely cause a photosensitivity. There is a theoretical risk of tar being carcinogenic because of absorption of polycyclic aromatic hydrocarbons.

Wood tars are obtained from the juniper tree, which on distillation produces Oil of Cade. This is used by some dermatological departments to treat scalp psoriasis. It would win the prize for the messiest preparation the author has ever seen prescribed!

Methotrexate

- Indication—psoriasis.
- NB. Dosage is weekly.
- No/minimal alcohol consumption.
- Haematological problems—marrow suppression, need to monitor FBC.
- Hepatic problems—fibrosis and cirrhosis.
- Monitor–LFTS, biochemical monitoring of type III prococcagen may replace liver biopsies.

Oral retinoids

- Common indications include very severe acne and psoriasis.
- Rarer indications—Darier's disease and pityriasis rubra pilaris.
- Acne—isotretinoin.
- Psoriasis—acitretin, has a long half-life.
- Oral retinoids are highly teratogenic.
- Effective contraception—during and 1 month after isotretinoin.
- Effective contraception—1 month before, during and 2 years after acitretin therapy.
- Side effects—hair loss and nosebleeds, sore lips, dryness of mucous membranes.
- Biochemical problems—can elevate lipids.

Phototherapy and photochemotherapy

- Indications—psoriasis, mycosis fungoides and atopic eczema.
- Increased risk—skin malignancies.
- Induced skin malignancies—related to type of therapy and cumulative doses.
- Relative risk—broad-band UVB < PUVA.
- Narrow-band UVB, more effective broad-band UVB.
- Skin ageing associated with PUVA.

Antibiotics

Topical antibiotics
Localized superficial infections can be treated using topical antibiotics, while systemic antibiotics are required if infection is more widespread. Topical fusidic acid or mupirocin are effective in most cases. Neomycin can cause a contact allergic dermatitis. There are a range of topical antibiotics to use in mild to moderate acne. These include clindamycin, erythromycin and tetracycline. They overcome the systemic side effects of oral therapy and they have a low potential to produce sensitivity. However, they can cause the development of bacterial resistance.

Systemic antibiotics

Systemic penicillin can be used to treat streptococcal infections. However, most *Staphylococcus aureus* infections are resistant to penicillin and require flucloxacillin. Erythromycin can be prescribed for patients allergic to penicillin. It has the advantage of treating both staphylococcal and streptococcal infections.

Systemic antibiotics, such as tetracycline and erythromycin, are used long-term to treat acne. Gastrointestinal disturbance is not uncommon. Broad-spectrum antibiotics can interfere with the efficacy of oral contraceptives and patients must be warned of possible interactions.

Systemic antibiotics		
Antibiotic	Dosage (adults)	Duration (days)
Penicillin	250–500 mg q.d.s.	5–10
Flucloxacillin	250–500 mg q.d.s.	5–10
Erythromycin	250–500 mg q.d.s.	7–14
Azithromycin	500 mg o.d.	3
Clarithromycin	250–500 mg b.d.	7–14
Ciprofloxacin	250–750 mg b.d.	5–10

Antiseptics

Hydrogen peroxide cream can be used to treat minor localized skin infections. Potassium permanganate soaks are useful in acute weeping situations, such as pompholyx, where secondary infection is common. Benzalkonium chloride is an antiseptic which has activity against Gram-positive bacteria. Using this in the long term can reduce the staphylococcal colonization of atopic eczema. However, antiseptics can be irritant, therefore one needs to use preparations combining an antiseptic with an emollient.

Useful tips for antiseptics:
- hydrogen peroxide cream for treating impetigo
- potassium permanganate soaks for treating pompholyx
- benzalkonium in combination with bath emollient for eczema.

Antifungals

Topical antifungals

Topical antifungals are the treatment of choice for minor fungal infections. When using topical antifungals important points are:

- nystatin is only effective against yeasts
- imidazoles are effective against yeasts and dermatophytes
- ketoconazole is highly effective against the yeast *Pityrosporum ovale*
- imidazoles are effective against yeasts, dermatophytes and some bacteria
- topical terbinafine is effective against yeasts and dermatophytes
- those who still favour Whitfield's Ointment should rub some in their own groin!

Oral antifungals

Oral antifungals are used to treat extensive skin infections and when hair or nails are involved. Griseofulvin is the oldest systemic antifungal, is fungistatic and only treats dermatophytes; it has largely been replaced by newer agents. Griseofulvin can interact with oral contraceptives. Terbinafine is a very effective fungicidal therapy for dermatophyte infections. Itraconazole is effective at treating both yeasts and dermatophyte infections. Ketoconazole is reserved for topical use, as systemic therapy can cause hepatic problems. Fluconazole can be used to treat both yeast and dermatophyte infections.

Caution is required prescribing systemic therapies for patients with hepatic and renal impairment. There are potential drug interactions and the data should be consulted for each individual drug. Oral antifungals should be avoided during pregnancy and while breastfeeding. Interestingly, griseofulvin carries warnings for males who want to father children.

Antivirals

Antivirals are sometimes used to treat herpes simplex and varicella zoster infections. As these are usually self-limiting conditions, it does not always seem necessary to prescribe medication. However, those who are immunosuppressed need urgent attention. Some topical antivirals are available over the counter to treat herpes simplex infections, and then it is the patient's decision.

Aciclovir is active against the herpes simplex and varicella zoster viruses. It is available in oral and topical formulations. Valaciclovir is the ester of aciclovir and acts as a prodrug, releasing aciclovir but needing less frequent oral administration. Penciclovir is used topically in similar situations to topical aciclovir. It has a prodrug famciclovir, which can be given orally in similar situations to oral aciclovir, but needs less frequent administration.

Scabicides and pediculocides

The first scabicide was sulphur which was thought to go back to Egyptian times. Benzyl benzoate is another old effective remedy, although skin irritation reduces its use. Because lindane takes such a long time to biodegrade its use could be detrimental to the environment. Chrysanthemums contain pyrethrum, and permethrin is a synthetic pyrethroid which is an ideal scabicide. It is of low toxicity and is cosmetically acceptable.

Head lice
To treat head lice one can use:
- malathion liquid
- carbaryl liquid
- permethrin cream rinse
- phenothrin lotion
- physical means.

To avoid a problem for asthmatic patients they should use aqueous preparations. Lotions have a longer contact time than shampoos. Because of anxiety over the safety of insecticide only those with active infection should be treated. Carbaryl has been associated with possible carcinogenicity when given orally long-term to rodents [47].

The team approach

The concept of a practice team continues to grow; gone are the days of the GP working in isolation. The team can provide comprehensive patient care, developing strategies to manage common chronic skin diseases within primary care. One partner within a practice may act as an in-house resource, helping with the diagnosis of patients with skin disease. An appropriately trained practice nurse could supervise the long-term care of patients with common dermatological problems.

The primary health care team

Practice nurse
Nurses have become actively involved in the management of asthma in primary care and there is no reason why they should not become involved in the management of atopic eczema. Helping patients to overcome skin disease improves their quality of life. Patients have often lost motivation and need the enthusiasm of the practice nurse to get them started. It is the correct usage of treatment which so often makes the difference between success and failure. Practice nurses can:
- demonstrate therapies
- perform compliance checks
- monitor therapies
- support patients.

The treatment plan for problems such as leg ulcers needs to be formulated by all the members of the team. The nurse is frequently the key person for a patient with a leg ulcer.

Health visitor
Health visitors are actively involved in health education. They see all new babies and hence their mothers. Health visitors should:
- educate on the treatment of nappy rash and atopic eczema
- dispel myths on diet and atopic eczema
- educate on the risks of skin cancer and sunlight.

Cosmetic camouflage service

This service can be more beneficial than trying multiple therapies which are of dubious benefit. Vascular lesions and vitiligo are two conditions which spring to mind.

Pharmacist

Many patients with minor skin problems seek the pharmacist's expertise. Pharmacists can advise on the appropriate application and storage of topical medication. Minor degrees of acne and eczema can be treated with over-the-counter products, and sometimes a medication is less expensive over the counter than a prescription charge. Holiday-makers need advice on sunscreens. All those involved in the treatment of skin disease should visit the local pharmacy. They should see how the creams and ointments they prescribe look, smell and spread.

Chiropodist

Patients with diabetes need good foot care. The chiropodist can manage children's verrucae and the elderly's callosities.

A key issue for the team—skin cancer

Melanoma is rare in childhood, but a major factor in its development in later life is sunburn in childhood. It is vital that the team give out this message using campaigns within their practice. It is essential that parents are taught to protect their children's skin. Children and young people should be encouraged to sit in the shade at times when sunlight is most intense, e.g. between 11 a.m. and 3 p.m. Being in water, e.g. swimming, does not protect people from sunlight.

There is a need to encourage the use of appropriate clothing and sunscreens. If clothing is held up to the light one can see how transparent it is. This reflects how effective it is at protecting from solar radiation. Patients should have some idea of their skin type, e.g. are they a red head who tend to burn easily? As medical students Barbara and I went off to Brighton one August Bank holiday, only to return to London with her feeling decidedly unwell and as red as a lobster! Sunscreens have to be of a high factor and applied frequently. Advice leaflets can help them with this.

CHAPTER 21

Guidelines

Guidelines can help foster the development of the concept of team work. Each member then feels that they are working with their colleagues to provide a uniform high standard of care. Guidelines exist for a number of common conditions including:

- atopic eczema
- psoriasis
- fungal nail disease
- management of leg ulcers.

Local guidelines should be developed from national guidelines by those who intend to implement them. They should be clear, concise and easy to follow. If only life was that simple!

Patient information

Leaflets

There are a whole range of sources of patient information leaflets, these include:

- British Association of Dermatologists
- patient support groups
- health education resource centres
- pharmaceutical companies
- inserts included with medication.

Organizations such as the British Association of Dermatologists, produce computer discs enabling practices to print leaflets as they require them. Some journals and pharmaceutical companies produce leaflets which can be photocopied. It is always worth personalizing a leaflet for each patient by writing points pertinent to that particular person on the leaflet. If one has the time it is worth trying to develop some of your own leaflets.

Modern technology

Videos have been produced which educate patients on how to use various therapies. CD-ROMs are now appearing on the scene, fulfilling similar functions, and these operate with a computer and a touch-sensitive screen.

22 Self-help

Patient self-help groups are playing an ever increasing part. They are an invaluable source of information for patients and doctors. The following is a list of self-help groups and other relevant organizations.

Acne Support Group, PO Box 230, Hayes, Middlesex UB4 9HW.

BACUP (skin cancer), 3 Bath Place, Rivington Street, London EC2A 3JR.

Behçet's Syndrome, 3 Church Close, Lambourn, Berkshire RG16 7PU.

Bullous Pemphigoid Support Group, PO Box 1059, Caterham, Surrey CR3 6ZU.

British Red Cross (provide a camouflage cosmetic service), 9 Grosvenor Crescent, London SW1X 7EJ.

Darier's Disease Support Group, PO Box 36, Milford Haven, Dyfed SA73 3YF.

Dystrophic Epidermolysis Bullosa Research Association (DEBRA), 13 Wellington Business Park, Duke's Ride, Crowthorne, Berkshire RG45 6LS.

Ehlers–Danlos Support Group, 1 Chandler Close, Richmond, North Yorkshire DL10 5QQ.

Hairline International, 1668 High Street, Knowle, Solihull B93 0LY.

Herpes Viruses Association, 41 North Road, London N7 9DP.

Ichthyosis Support Group, 562 Workingham Road, Earley, Reading.

Tissue Viability Society, Glanville Centre, Salisbury District Hospital, Salisbury, Wiltshire SP2 8BJ.

Lupus UK, 1 Eastern Road, Romford, Essex RM1 3NH.

Lymphoedema Support Network, St Luke's Crypt, Sydney Street, London SW3 6NH.

For professional enquiries: British Lymphoma Support Group, Administration Centre, PO Box 1059, Caterham, Surrey CR3 6ZU.

National Eczema Society, 163 Eversholt Street, London NW1 1BU.

Neurofibromatosis Association, 82 London Road, Kingston-upon-Thames, Surrey KT2 6PX.

Pemphigus Vulgaris Network, Flat C, 26 St German's Road, London SE23 1RJ.

Pseudoxanthoma Elasticum Support Group, 15 Mead Close, Marlow, Buckinghamshire SL7 1HR.

CHAPTER 22

Psoriasis Association, 7 Milton Street, Northampton NN2 7JG.

Raynaud's and Scleroderma Association, 112 Crewe Road, Alsager, Cheshire ST7 2JA.

Sun Know How Campaign, Health Education Authority, Hamilton House, Mabledon Place, London WC1H 9TX.

Tuberous Sclerosis Association, Little Barnsley Farm, Catshill, Bromsgrove, Worcestershire B61 0NQ.

Vitiligo Society, 19 Fitzroy Square, London W1P 5HQ.

Postscript

I hope you have found this little book helpful and I have stimulated your interest in skin disease in primary care. Without Barbara's help I would never have put pen to paper; I hope the trees will forgive me! Finally I would like to thank Dr A. Carmichael for his wonderful teaching and contributing some of his slides to this book.

References

1 Office of Population Census and Surveys. *Morbidity Statistics from General Practice. Fourth National Study*, 1991–92: 54–5.
2 Burge S., Clover G. & Lester R. *Simple Skin Surgery.* Blackwell Science, Oxford, 1996.
3 Lawrence C. *An Introduction to Dermatological Surgery.* Blackwell Science, Oxford, 1997.
4 Sladden M.J. & Graham-Brown R. How many referrals to dermatology outpatients are really necessary? *J R Soc Med* 1989; **82**: 437–8.
5 Basarab T., Munn S.E. & Rusell Jones R. Diagnostic accuracy and appropriateness of referrals to a dermatology out-patient clinic. *Br J Dermatol* 1996; **135**: 70–1.
6 Cunliffe W. Acne and unemployment. *Br J Dermatol* 1986; **115**: 386.
7 Finlay A.Y. The scaly patient. *Dermatol Prac* 1987; **5**: 28.
8 Williams H., Burney P., Pembroke A. & Hayes R. The UK working party's diagnostic criteria for atopic dermatitis. III. Independent hospital validation. *Br J Dermatol* 1994; **131**: 406–17.
9 MacKie R. Clinical recognition of early invasive malignant melanoma. Looking for changes in size, shape and colour is successful. *BMJ* 1990; **301**: 1005–6.
10 Fitzpatrick T., Rhodes A. & Sober A. Primary malignant melanoma of the skin: the call for action to identify persons at risk: to discover precursor lesions: to detect early melanomas. *Pigment Cell* 1988; **9**: 110–17.
11 British Society for Dermatological Surgery. *Guidelines for Surgical Management of Common Skin Conditions in General Practice.* Personal Communication, 1994.
12 Khorshid S., Pinney E. & Newton Bishop J. Melanoma excised by general practitioners in North-East Thames region, England. *Br J Dermatol* 1998; **138**: 412–17.
13 Hunter D. Controversies in the management of malignant melanoma. *Br J Hospital Med* 1993; **49**: 174–80.
14 Del Mar B. & Green A. Aid to diagnosis of melanoma in primary care. *BMJ* 1995; **310**: 492–5.
15 Berth-Jones J. Six Area, Six Sign Atopic Dermatitis (SASSAD) severity score: a simple system for monitoring disease activity in atopic dermatitis. *Br J Dermatol* 1996; **135** (Suppl. 48): 25–30.

16 Brazier J.E., Harper R., Jones N.M. *et al.* Validating the SF-36 health survey questionnaire new outcome measures for primary care. *BMJ* 1992; **305**: 160–4.

17 The Children's Dermatology Life Quality Index (CDLQI). Initial validation and practical use. *Br J Dermtol* 1995; **132**: 942–9.

18 Finlay A.Y. & Khan G.K. Dermatology Life Quality Index (DLQI): a simple practical measure for routine clinical use. *Clin Exp Dermatol* 1994; **19**: 210–16.

19 Harlow D., Poyner T., Finlay A.Y. & Dykes P.J. High impairment of quality of life of adults with skin diseases in primary care. *Br J Dermatol* 1998; **139** (Suppl. 51): 15.

20 Motley R.J. & Finlay A.Y. Practical use of a disability index in the routine management of acne. *Clin Exp Dermatol* 1992; **17**: 1–3.

21 Finlay A.Y. & Kelly S.E. Psoriasis — an index of disability. *Clin Exp Dermatol* 1987; **12**: 8–11.

22 Lawson V, Lewis Jones MS, Finlay AY *et al.* The family impact of childhood atopic dermatitis: the Dermatitis Family Impact questionnaire. *BJD* 1998; **138**: 107–11.

23 Osbourne J.E., Bourke J.F., Holder J. *et al.* The effect of the introduction of a pigmented lesion clinic on the interval between referral by family practitioner and attendance at hospital. *Br J Dermatol* 1998; **138**: 418–21.

24 Gough A., Chapman S., Wagstaff K., Emery P. & Elias E. Minocycline induced autoimmune hepatitis and systemic lupus erythematosus-like syndrome. *BMJ* 1996; **312**: 169–72.

25 Ferner R.E. & Moss C. Minocycline for acne. *BMJ* 1996; **312**: 138.

26 Cotterill J.A. & Cunliffe WJ. Suicide in dermatological patients. *Br J Dermatol* 1997; **137**: 246–50.

27 Macfadden J., Noble W. & Camp R. Superantigenic exotoxin secreting potential of Staphylococci isolated from atopic eczematous skin. *Br J Dermatol* 1993; **128**: 631–2.

28 Molloy H.F., LaMont-Gregory E., Idzikowski C. & Ryan T.J. Overheating in bed as an important factor in common dermatoses. *Int J. Dermatol* 1993; **32**: 668–72.

29 McHenry M., Williams H. & Bingham E. Management of atopic eczema. *BMJ* 1995; **310**: 843–7.

30 Poyner T. Current management of psoriasis. Recommendations for initial management. *J Dermatol Treatment* 1997; **8**: 27–55.

31 Razicka T. & Lorenz B. Comparison of calcipotriol monotherapy and a combination of calcipotriol and betamethasone valerate after 2 weeks, treatment with calcipotriol in the topical therapy of psoriasis vulgaris: a multicentre, double-blind, randomised study. *Br J Dermatol* 1998; **138**: 254–8.

32 Alpsoy E. & Cetin L. Is the efficacy of topical corticosteroid therapy for psoriasis vulgaris enhanced by concurrent moclobemide therapy? *Am J Dermatol* 1998; **38**: 197–200.

33 Williams R. Guidelines for management of patients with psoriasis. *BMJ* 1991; **303**: 829–35.
34 Ingram J.T. The approach to psoriasis. *British Medical Journal* 1953; ii: 591–4.
35 Finlay A.Y. Treatment of onychomycosis. In: *Skin Therapy* (R. Marks & W.J. Cunliffe eds). London: Martin Dunitz, 1994.
36 Denning D.W., Evans E.G.V. & Kibbler C.C. Fungal nail disease: a guide to good practice (report of a Working Group of the British Society for Medical Mycology). *BMJ* 1995; **311**: 1277–81.
37 Massing A. & Epstein W. Natural history of warts: a two year study. *Arch Dermatol* 1963; **87**: 306–10.
38 Cork M. Economic considerations in the treatment of psoriasis. *Dermatol Prac* 1993; **1**: 673–7.
39 Maurice P. & Saiham E. Topical steroid requirement in inflammatory skin conditions. *Br J Clin Pract* 1985; **39**: 441.
40 Long C.C. & Finlay A.Y. The fingertip unit: a new practical measure. *Clin Exp Dermatol* 1991; **18**: 444–6.
41 Long C., Mills C. & Finlay A. A practical guide to topical therapy for children. *Br J Dermatol* 1998; **138**: 293–6.
42 Buxton P.K. *ABC of Dermatology* London: BMA, 1988: 16.
43 Coulson I. Topical steroids for skin disease. *Dermatol Prac* 1996; **4**(2): 5–9.
44 Poyner T.F., Hughes J.W., Dass B.K. *et al.* Long term treatment of chronic plaque psoriasis with calcipotriol. *J Dermatol Treat* 1993; **4**: 173–7.
45 Veien N.K., Bjerke J.R. & Rossmann-Ringdahl I. *et al.* Once daily treatment of psoriasis with tacalcitol compared with twice daily treatment with calcipotriol. *Br J Dermatol* 1997; **137**: 581–6.
46 Weinstein G.D., Krueger G.G., Lowe N.J. *et al.* Tazarotene gel, a new retinoid, for topical therapy of psoriasis: vehicle-controlled study of safety, efficacy and duration of therapeutic effect. *J Am Acad Dermatol* 1997; **37**: 85–92.
47 Department of Health. *Carbaryl.* London: Department of Health, 1995 (Professional Letter: PL/CMO(95)4, PL/CNO(95)3).

Index

Page numbers in *italics* indicate figures

abscess, 19
absorption, drug, 145
acanthosis nigricans, 67, 68, 71, 72
aciclovir, 140, 141, 161
acitretin, 158
acne, 1, 25, 26, 27
  employment problems, 15
  grading, 105
  indications for referral, 115
  management, 109–15
  systemic therapy, 111–13
  topical therapy, 110, 111
acrivastine, 154
actinic dermatitis, chronic, 32
actinic keratosis, 12, 31, 32, 80, 92
adapalene, 156
alcohol consumption, 15
allergic contact dermatitis, 4, 58
  face, 24, 31
  feet, 81, 83
  flexures, 70
  hands, 76, 77, 79
  lower legs, 59, 60
  patch testing, 101–2
alopecia
  androgenetic, 36, 132
  areata, 36, 84, 86, 131
amorolfine, 137
anal irritation (pruritus ani), 73, 130
angioedema, 23–4, 102, 133
angiomas, 12
ankle/brachial pressure ratio, 103–4
anthralin (dithranol), 126, 156–7
antibiotics, 158–9
  in acne, 110, 111–12
  in cellulitis, 135
  in eczema, 118
  infected leg ulcers, 144
  systemic, 159
  topical, 110, 111, 158
antifungals, 160
  oral, 136, 137, 160
  topical, 136, 137, 160
antihistamines, 154–5
  non-sedative, 133, 154–5

  sedative, 155
antimalarials, 116
antiseptics, 159
antivirals, 140–1, 160–1
aqueous cream, 150
asteatotic eczema, 6, 37, 59, *60*, 122
athlete's foot *see* tinea, pedis
atopic eczema, 3, 39–41
  face, 22–3, 31
  flexures, 68, 70
  management, 117, 118–21
Auspitz's sign, 42
autoimmune diseases, 67
azelaic acid, 110, 111, *114*
azithromycin, 159

bacterial infections, 118
  investigations, 99
  management, 135, 158–9
balanitis, 73
basal cell carcinoma (BCC), 12, 47, 93–4
basal cell papillomas (seborrhoeic warts), 11, 32, 89–90
bathing, in atopic eczema, 119
benzalkonium chloride, 159
benzoyl peroxide, 110, 111, *114*
benzyl benzoate, 161
betamethasone valerate, 151
biopsy, 104
blistering rashes, 56–8, 80, 83
blood tests, 102
Bowen's disease, 47, 60, 93
bulla, 19
bullous diseases, inflammatory, 59

calcipotriol, 126, *128*, 155
callosities, 89
Candida infections
  genitalia, 73, 75
  hands, 79
  management, 136
  nails, 84, 86

carbaryl, 161
carbuncle, 19
CD-ROMs, patient information, 164
cellulitis
    lower legs, 59, 60, 61, 62
    management, 135
cetirizine, 133, 154
chickenpox, 57, 118
children
    facial rashes, 22–3
    sunburn prevention, 163
chiropodist, 163
chloasma, 32, 115–16
chlorpheniramine, 155
chondrodermatitis nodularis chronica
        helicis, 31, 91
ciprofloxacin, 159
clarithromycin, 159
clindamycin, 110, 158
clobetasol propionate, 151
clobetasone butyrate, 151
clotrimazole, 136
cold sores see herpes simplex
        infections
colour, 20
comedones, 25, 27, 32
contact dermatitis, 3–4, 47
    allergic see allergic contact
        dermatitis
    flexures, 68
    hands, 77–9
    irritant, 3, 77–9, 121–2
    management, 121–2
corticosteroids see steroids
cosmetic camouflage service, 163
creams, 148
crusts, 18
cryosurgery, 139, 140
cutaneous horn, 92
cyclosporin, 121, 154
cyproterone acetate, 113

dandruff, 34, 41
dapsone, 116
Darier's disease, 7
dermatitis see eczema
dermatitis herpetiformis, 59, 104
dermatofibroma, 11, 90
dermatology life quality index
        (DLQI), 106
dermatomyositis, 67, 76
dermatophyte infections see tinea
dermatosis papulosa nigra, 32

dermographism, 53, 55
diabetes mellitus, 65–7
Dianette, 113, 114
discoid eczema, 5, 41, 42, 47
    management, 117, 124
discoid lupus erythematosus, 31, 109,
        116
dithranol, 126, 128, 156–7
Doppler ultrasound, 103–4
doxycycline, 112
drug eruptions, 9, 51, 57–8
dry skin, 37

ears, 23, 31
eczema, 2–7, 38–41
    endogenous, 2, 38
    exogenous, 2, 38
    facial, 22–3, 117
    flexural, 70, 117
    hand see hand eczema
    herpeticum, 118
    infections and, 118
    management, 117–24
    severity scoring, 105
    see also specific types
emollients, 126, 150–1
emulsifying ointment, 150–1
epidermoid cyst, 90–1
erosion, 18
erysipelas, 24–5, 135
erythema, 18, 20
    chronicum migrans, 56
    multiforme, 57–8
    nodosum, 59, 60–1
    toxic, 55
erythrasma, 68, 69–70, 101, 135
erythroderma, 55
erythromycin
    systemic, 111, 112, 115, 135, 159
    topical, 110, 158
examination, 16–21
excoriations, 18
exudate, 18

face, 22–33
    childhood rashes, 22–3
    excessive hair, 33
    management of rashes, 109–16
    mature, 32
    pigmentation abnormalities, 32
    red, in adults, 23–32
famciclovir, 141, 161

family history, 15
feet, 80, 81–3
fexofenadine, 133
finasteride, 132
fingertip units (FTU), 147
fissures, 18
flexural rashes, 68–75, 130–1
flucloxacillin, 115, 122, 135, 144, 159
fluconazole, 160
fluocortolone, 151
folliculitis, 28
formulations, 147–9
fungal infections
    flexures, 69
    investigations, 99–101
    management, 130, 136–9
    nails, 84, 85, 137
    see also Candida infections; tinea
furuncle, 19
fusidic acid, 135, 158

gels, 148
genitalia, 73–5
glutaraldehyde, 140
granuloma annulare, 53, 56, 67
    hands, 76, 77, 79
    management, 133
griseofulvin, 137, 138, 160
guidelines, 164

Hailey–Hailey disease, 68
hair loss, 34–6
    diffuse, 34–6
    localized, 36
halcinonide, 151
hand eczema, 76–7, 117
    industrial, 77–9
    management, 122
hand-foot-and-mouth disease, 80, 83
hands, 76–80
head lice, 34, 141–2, 161
health visitor, 162
Henoch–Schönlein purpura, 63
herpes simplex infections, 28, 29
    in atopic eczema, 41, 118
    genital, 73, 75
    investigations, 100
    management, 140–1
herpes zoster, 57, 141
hidradenitis suppurativa, 68, 71, 72, 130
hirsutism, 33, 132

history, clinical, 14–16
horn, cutaneous, 92
house dust mite, 119–21
hydrocortisone, 151, 152
hydrogen peroxide cream, 159
hydroxychloroquine, 116
hyperhidrosis, 81, 131
hyperkeratotic eczema, 76
hypomelanosis, guttate, 50, 51

ichthyoses, 37, 38
imidazole, 138
immunodeficiency, 141
immunofluorescence, 104
immunology, 102
immunosuppressants, 153–4
impetigo, 10, 23, 24, 57
    management, 135
industrial hand dermatitis, 77–9
infants, eczema, 22, 23
infections see skin infections
infestations, 141–2
inflammatory bullous diseases, 59
information, patient, 164
intertrigo, 68, 69, 136
investigations, 99–105
irritant contact dermatitis, 3, 77–9, 121–2
isotretinoin, 113, 156, 158
itch, 15, 53
    generalized, 37, 103
    –scratch cycle, 119
itraconazole, 136, 137, 138, 160

juvenile plantar dermatosis, 81, 82, 124
juvenile spring eruption, 23, 31, 32

Kaposi's varicelliform eruption, 41
keloids, 91
keratoacanthoma, 92
keratolysis, pitted, 81–3, 135
ketoconazole, 136, 137, 160
knuckle pads, 76
Koebner's phenomenon, 17, 18, 87

larva migrans, 81
leaflets, patient information, 164
legs, lower, 59–63, 64
leg ulcers, 13, 63–7

leg ulcers (Cont.)
  chronic venous, 63, 65
  ischaemic, 65–7
  management, 143–4
lentigines, 32, 80
lentigo maligna, 96
leukoplakia, 75
lice, head, 34, 141–2, 161
lichenification, 18
lichen planus, 8, 44, 45, 47
  genitalia, 75
  nails, 84, 86
  treatment, 129
lichen sclerosus et atrophicus, 75, 131
lichen simplex, 6, 47
  flexures, 68, 70
  management, 124
lindane, 161
lipoma, 91
loratadine, 133, 154
lotions, 148
lupus erythematosus
  discoid, 31, 109, 116
  systemic, 31
lupus pernio, 27
lymecycline, 112
Lyme disease, 56

macule, 18
malathion, 161
malignancy, 67
massage, 119
measurement, dermatological, 105–6
melanoma, 11, 13, 94–8, 163
  acral lentiginous, 98
  amelanotic, 96
  investigations, 104
  lentigo maligna, 96
  nails, 84–6
  nodular, 96, 97
  secondary, 53
  superficial spreading, 96, 97
melasma, 32, 51, 115–16
methotrexate, 157
metronidazole, 144
miconazole, 135
milia, 91
minocycline, 111—12, 114
minoxidil, topical, 132
molluscum contagiosum, 10, 89, 140
mometasone, 151
morphoea, 50, 51, 134
mupirocin, 135, 158

mycosis fungoides, 44, 47
myxoedema, pretibial, 60

naevi, 11
nails, 84–6, 132
  clippings, 100
  fungal infections, 84, 85, 137
  in psoriasis, 84, 85, 86, 127
nappy rash, 71, 122, 136
necrobiosis lipoidica, 60, 61, 62, 67
necrotizing fasciitis, 61
neomycin, 158
neurofibromatosis, 53
nicotinamide, 110
Nikolsky's sign, 59
nodules, 19, 52–6
nystatin, 160

occupational disorders, 15, 77–9, 121
Oil of Cade, 157
oily cream, 150
ointments, 148
onycholysis, 84
onychomycosis, 84, 137
orf, 79, 80
otitis externa, 30

paints, 148
papules, 19, 52–6
paronychia, 19
  acute, 135
  chronic, 84, 136, 137
paste, 149
patches, 18, 50–1
patch testing, 101–2
patient information, 164
pediculocides, 161
pemphigoid, 59, 104
  gestationis, 59, 67
pemphigus, 59, 104
penciclovir, 140, 161
penicillin, 135, 144, 159
penile rashes, 75
perioral dermatitis, 27, 115
permethrin, 142, 161
persistent superficial dermatitis, 44, 45
pets, 120
pharmacist, 163
phenothrin, 161
photochemotherapy, 158

photodermatoses *see* solar-related
  conditions
photography, 105
phototherapy, 158
phytophotodermatitis, 58
pigmentation, abnormal, 32, 51
pilar cyst, 90–1
pitted keratolysis, 81–3, 135
pityriasis
  alba, 22, 51, 124
  lichenoides, 44, 45
  rosea, 8, 42, 44, 45, *46*
    treatment, 129
  rubra pilaris, 9
  versicolor, 51, 101, 136
Pityrosporum yeast, 41, 51, 136
plaques, 18
  itchy, 47
  localized, 47–51
podophyllum, 140
polymorphic eruption of pregnancy,
  67
polymorphic light eruption, 27, 32,
  116
pompholyx, 5, 76, 80, 122
porphyria cutanea tarda, 80
potassium permanganate soaks, 147,
  159
powders, 149
practice nurse, 162
pregnancy, 67
prick test, 102
primary health care team, 162–3
prurigo, nodular, 53
pruritic urticarial papules and plaques
  of pregnancy, 67
pruritus *see* itch
pruritus ani, 73, 130
psoriasis, 8, 42, 43, 47
  facial, 28–30, 127
  flexural, 68, 71, 126–7
  guttate, 42, 44, 126
  hands and feet, 76, 81
  indications for referral, 127
  management, 125–9
  nails, 84, *85*, 86, 127
  penile, 75
  plaque, 42, *43*, 44, 126
  pustular, hands and feet, 80, 81,
    126
  scalp, 34, *35*, 125
  severity scoring, 105
  systemic therapy, 127–9
  topical therapy, 126

psychological problems, 15, 113
purpura, 20
pustule, 19
pyogenic granuloma, 91

quality of life
  measurement, 105–6
  in psoriasis, 127

referrals, 106–7
retinoids, 156
  oral, 113, 158
  topical, 110, 111, 156
rhinophyma, 27, *28*
ringworm *see* tinea
rosacea, 2, 25, *26*, 27, 115

salicylic acid, 139, 140, 154
sarcoid, 27, 31, 53
scabicides, 142, 161
scabies, 11, 52, 53, 75, 76
  Norwegian, 53, 76
  treatment, 142
scalded skin syndrome, 57
scale, 18
scalp, 34–6, 131–2
scaly plaques, localized, 47
scaly rashes, 38–47, *48*
seborrhoeic eczema
  adult, 5, 28–30, 31, 41, 124
  flexures, 68, 70
  infantile, 5, 22, *23*, 122
  scalp, 34, *35*
  treatment, 117, 118, 124, 136
seborrhoeic warts (basal cell
    papillomas), 11, 32, 89–90
self-help groups, patient, 165–6
shampoo, 148
shingles (herpes zoster), 57, 141
skin infections, 9–11
  blistering, 57
  in eczema, 118
  management, 135–42
skin tumours, 11–13, 87–98
  benign, 11–12, 87–92
  malignant (cancer), 11, 12–13,
    93–8, 163
skin types, 105
smoking, 15
soaks, 147
solar keratosis *see* actinic keratosis

solar-related conditions, 30, 31–2, 80
  prevention, 163
  treatment, 116
squamous cell carcinoma, 12, 94
Staphylococcus aureus, 57, 118, 135
stasis eczema *see* venous eczema
steroids
  oral, 153
  topical, 117, 151–3
    potency, 151–2
    side effects, 152–3
    site of application, 152
Streptococcus pyogenes, 135
strimmer (weed wacker's) dermatitis,
    60, 63
subungual haematoma, 84
suicide, 113
swabs, 99, 100
Sweet's disease, 53
sycosis barbae, 28, 29, 115
symmetrical rash, 49
systemic lupus erythematosus, 31

tacalcitol, 128, 155
tar, 126, 157
tazarotene, 156
team, primary health care, 162–3
telangiectasia, 20, 79
terbinafine, 136, 137, 138, 160
terfenadine, 154, 155
tetracycline, 111, 112, 114, 158, 159
threadworms, 73
thyroid disease, 67
tinea, 47
  capitis, 36, 101, 137
  corporis, 44, 47
  cruris, 69, 70, 136
  face, 31
  flexures, 68, 69
  hands, 76, 79
  id reaction, 79
  incognito, 14, 99
  nails, 84, 85, 86
  pedis (athlete's foot), 10, 80, 81,
    136
  treatment, 136–9
topical therapy, 145–9
  duration, 145–6
  formulations, 147–9
  health economics, 146
  volumes, 146–7
toxic epidermal necrolysis, 57

toxic erythema, 55
tretinoin, 156
trichotillomania, 36
trimethoprim, 112, 114

ulcers, 18
  leg *see* leg ulcers
urea, 154
urticaria, 9, 53–4, 55
  acute, 53–4
  chronic, 54
  management, 133
  solar, 116

valaciclovir, 141, 161
varicose eczema *see* venous eczema
vasculitis, 60, 63
venous eczema (varicose eczema), 6, 7,
    59, 60
  management, 117, 124, 143
verrucae, 79, 89, 139–40
videos, patient information, 164
viral infections, 139–41
vitamin A derivatives, 126, 156
  see also retinoids
vitamin D derivatives, 125, 126,
    155–6
vitiligo, 50, 51, 101, 134
vulval rashes, 73

warts
  filiform, 87, 88, 89
  genital, 75, 140
  mosaic, 89, 140
  plane, 87, 88, 89, 140
  seborrhoeic (basal cell papillomas),
    11, 32, 89–90
  treatment, 139–40
  viral, 9, 10, 79, 87–9
weals, 18, 52–6
weed wacker's dermatitis, 60, 63
wet wraps, 119, 120
Wickham's striae, 44
Wood's light, 100–1

xanthoma, eruptive, 53

yeast infections, 136